T0227246

COVID-19 in the Geriatric Patient

Editor

FRANCESCO LANDI

CLINICS IN GERIATRIC MEDICINE

www.geriatric.theclinics.com

August 2022 • Volume 38 • Number 3

ELSEVIER

1600 John F. Kennedy Boulevard ● Suite 1800 ● Philadelphia, Pennsylvania, 19103-2899

http://www.theclinics.com

CLINICS IN GERIATRIC MEDICINE Volume 38, Number 3
August 2022 ISSN 0749–0690, ISBN-13: 978-0-323-96130-1

Editor: Taylor Hayes
Developmental Editor: Hannah Almira Lopez

Clinics in Geriatric Medicine (ISSN 0749-0690) is published quarterly by Elsevier Inc., 360 Park Avenue South, New York, NY 10010-1710. Months of issue are February, May, August, and November. Business and Editorial Offices: 1600 John F. Kennedy Blvd., Suite 1800, Philadelphia, PA 191023-2899. Periodicals postage paid at New York, NY, and additional mailing offices. Subscription prices are $303.00 per year (US individuals), $901.00 per year (US institutions), $100.00 per year (US & Canadian student/resident), $330.00 per year (Canadian individuals), $928.00 per year (Canadian institutions), $431.00 per year (international individuals), $928.00 per year (international institutions), and $195.00 per year (international student/resident). Foreign air speed delivery is included in all *Clinics* subscription prices. All prices are subject to change without notice. POSTMASTER: Send address changes to *Clinics in Geriatric Medicine,* Elsevier Health Sciences Division, Subscription Customer Service, 3251 Riverport Lane, Maryland Heights, MO 63043. **Telephone: 1-800-654-2452 (U.S. and Canada); 314-447-8871 (outside U.S. and Canada). Fax: 314-447-8029. E-mail:** journalscustomerservice-usa@elsevier.com **(for print support) or** journalsonlinesupport-usa@elsevier.com **(for online support).**

Reprints. For copies of 100 or more, of articles in this publication, please contact the Commercial Reprints Department, Elsevier Inc., 360 Park Avenue South, New York, New York 10010-1710. Tel.: 212-633-3874; Fax: 212-633-3820, E-mail: reprints@elsevier.com.

Clinics in Geriatric Medicine is covered in *MEDLINE/PubMed (Index Medicus), EMBASE/Excerpta Medica, Current Contents/Clinical Medicine (CC/CM),* and the *Cumulative Index to Nursing & Allied Health Literature.*

Contributors

EDITOR

FRANCESCO LANDI, MD, PhD
Associate Professor of Internal Medicine, Department of Geriatrics, Neurosciences and Orthopaedics, Catholic University of the Sacred Heart, Geriatric Department, Gemelli Against COVID-19 Post-acute Care Study Group, Fondazione Policlinico Universitario Agostino Gemelli IRCCS, Department of Translational and Precision Medicine, Sapienza University of Rome, Center for Geriatric Medicine (Ce.M.I.), Università Cattolica del Sacro Cuore, Rome, Italy

AUTHORS

MARIA CHIARA AGNITELLI, MD
Fondazione Policlinico Universitario Agostino Gemelli, IRCSS, Rome, Italy

FRANCES BATCHELOR, B App Scl, GradDipEd, MHS, PhD
Department of Physiotherapy, The University of Melbourne, Melbourne, Victoria, Australia; National Ageing Research Institute (NARI), Parkville, Australia; School of Nursing and Midwifery, Deakin University, Burwood, Victoria, Australia

JÜRGEN M. BAUER, MD, PhD
Center for Geriatric Medicine, Heidelberg University, Agaplesion Bethanien Hospital, Heidelberg, Germany

MARION BAZIARD, MD
Gerontopole of Toulouse, Institute on Aging, Toulouse University Hospital (CHU Toulouse), Toulouse, France

ANDREA BELLIENI, MD
Geriatrician, Center for Geriatric Medicine, Fondazione Policlinico Universitario Agostino Gemelli IRCCS, Rome, Italy

FRANCESCA BENVENUTO, MD
Gemelli Against COVID-19 Post-acute Care Study Group, Fondazione Policlinico Universitario Agostino Gemelli IRCCS, Rome, Italy

ROBERTO BERNABEI, MD
Gemelli Against COVID-19 Post-acute Care Study Group, Fondazione Policlinico Universitario Agostino Gemelli IRCCS, Rome, Italy

ALESSANDRA BIZZARRO, MD
Gemelli Against COVID-19 Post-acute Care Study Group, Fondazione Policlinico Universitario Agostino Gemelli IRCCS, Rome, Italy

GIULIA BRAMATO, MD
Gemelli Against COVID-19 Post-acute Care Study Group, Fondazione Policlinico Universitario Agostino Gemelli IRCCS, Rome, Italy

STEFANO CACCIATORE, MD
Physician, Fondazione Policlinico Universitario Agostino Gemelli IRCCS, Rome, Italy

RICCARDO CALVANI, PhD
Researcher, Center for Geriatric Medicine, Fondazione Policlinico Universitario Agostino Gemelli IRCCS, Rome, Italy

ANGELO CARFÌ, MD
Gemelli Against COVID-19 Post-acute Care Study Group, Centro Medicina dell'Invecchiamento, Fondazione Policlinico Universitario Agostino Gemelli IRCCS, Rome, Italy

LIANG-KUNG CHEN, MD, PhD
Center for Healthy Longevity and Aging Sciences, National Yang Ming Chiao Tung University, Center for Geriatrics and Gerontology, Taipei Veterans General Hospital, Taipei Municipal Gan-Dau Hospital (Managed by Taipei Veterans General Hospital), Taipei, Taiwan

ENEA CHISCI, MD
Physician, Fondazione Policlinico Universitario Agostino Gemelli IRCCS, Rome, Italy

FRANCESCA CICIARELLO, MD
Gemelli Against COVID-19 Post-acute Care Study Group, Geriatrician, Fondazione Policlinico Universitario Agostino Gemelli IRCCS, Geriatrician, Department of Geriatrics and Orthopedics, Università Cattolica del Sacro Cuore, Rome, Italy

HÉLIO JOSÉ COELHO-JÚNIOR, PhD
Researcher, Department of Geriatrics and Orthopedics, Università Cattolica del Sacro Cuore, Rome, Italy

ADELAIDE DE MAULEON, MD
Gerontopole of Toulouse, Institute on Aging, Toulouse University Hospital (CHU Toulouse), Toulouse, France

ANTONELLA DI PAOLA, Psy.D
Gemelli Against COVID-19 Post-acute Care Study Group, Fondazione Policlinico Universitario Agostino Gemelli IRCCS, Rome, Italy

ESTELLE DUBUS, MD
Gerontopole of Toulouse, Institute on Aging, Toulouse University Hospital (CHU Toulouse), Toulouse, France

GUSTAVO DUQUE, MD, PhD
Australian Institute for Musculoskeletal Science (AIMSS), Department of Medicine, The University of Melbourne and Western Health, St Albans, Victoria, Australia

MASSIMO FANTONI, MD
Gemelli Against COVID-19 Post-acute Care Study Group, Fondazione Policlinico Universitario Agostino Gemelli IRCCS, Rome, Italy

ANTONELLA GALLO, MD
Fondazione Policlinico Universitario Agostino Gemelli, IRCSS, Rome, Italy

VINCENZO GALLUZZO, MD
Geriatrician, Fondazione Policlinico Universitario Agostino Gemelli IRCCS, Rome, Italy

STEFAN GRUND, MD, MaHM
Center for Geriatric Medicine, Heidelberg University, Agaplesion Bethanien Hospital, Heidelberg, Germany

FEI-YUAN HSIAO, PhD
Graduate Institute of Clinical Pharmacy, College of Medicine, School of Pharmacy, College of Medicine, Department of Pharmacy, National Taiwan University, Taipei, Taiwan

FRANCESCA IBBA, MD
Fondazione Policlinico Universitario Agostino Gemelli, IRCSS, Rome, Italy

DELFINA JANIRI, MD
Gemelli Against COVID-19 Post-acute Care Study Group, Fondazione Policlinico Universitario Agostino Gemelli IRCCS, Rome, Italy

FRANCESCO LANDI, MD, PhD
Associate Professor of Internal Medicine, Department of Geriatrics, Neurosciences and Orthopaedics, Catholic University of the Sacred Heart, Geriatric Department, Gemelli Against COVID-19 Post-acute Care Study Group, Fondazione Policlinico Universitario Agostino Gemelli IRCCS, Department of Translational and Precision Medicine, Sapienza University of Rome, Center for Geriatric Medicine (Ce.M.I.), Università Cattolica del Sacro Cuore, L.go F. Vito 1, Rome, Italy

OLGA LAOSA, PhD, MD
Clinical Pharmacologist, CIBER of Frailty and Healthy Aging (CIBERFES), Institute of Health Carlos III, Geriatric Research Group, Biomedical Research Foundation at Getafe University Hospital, Madrid, Spain

ALESSANDRA LAURIA, MD
Gemelli Against COVID-19 Post-acute Care Study Group, Fondazione Policlinico Universitario Agostino Gemelli IRCCS, Rome, Italy

WEI-JU LEE, MD, PhD
Center for Healthy Longevity and Aging Sciences, National Yang Ming Chiao Tung University, Taipei, Taiwan; Department of Family Medicine, Taipei Veterans General Hospital Yuanshan Branch, Yi-Lan, Taiwan

MARIA SANDRINA LEONE, MD
Physician, Fondazione Policlinico Universitario Agostino Gemelli IRCCS, Rome, Italy

CHIH-KUANG LIANG, MD, PhD
Center for Healthy Longevity and Aging Sciences, National Yang Ming Chiao Tung University, Taipei, Taiwan; Center for Geriatrics and Gerontology, Kaohsiung Veterans General Hospital, Kaohsiung, Taiwan

NOEMI MACEROLA, MD
Fondazione Policlinico Universitario Agostino Gemelli, IRCSS, Rome, Italy

EMANUELE MARZETTI, MD, PhD
Associate Professor of Internal Medicine and Geriatrics, Center for Geriatric Medicine, Orthogeriatric Unit, Geriatrician, Fondazione Policlinico Universitario Agostino Gemelli IRCCS, Department of Geriatrics and Orthopedics, Università Cattolica del Sacro Cuore, L.go F. Vito 1, Rome, Italy

LIN-CHIEH MENG, BS, PHARM
Graduate Institute of Clinical Pharmacy, College of Medicine

MASSIMO MONTALTO, MD, PhD
Fondazione Policlinico Universitario Agostino Gemelli, IRCSS, Università Cattolica del Sacro Cuore, Rome, Italy

ROSSELLA MONTENERO, MD
Physician, Fondazione Policlinico Universitario Agostino Gemelli IRCCS, Rome, Italy

MONTSERRAT MONTES-IBARRA, MSc
PhD Student, Human Nutrition Research Unit, Department of Agricultural, Food, and Nutritional Science, University of Alberta, Edmonton, Alberta, Canada

CELESTE AMBRA MURACE, MD
Fondazione Policlinico Universitario Agostino Gemelli, IRCSS, Rome, Italy

CAMILA L.P. OLIVEIRA, PhD
Postdoctoral Fellow, Human Nutrition Research Unit, Department of Agricultural, Food, and Nutritional Science, University of Alberta, Edmonton, Alberta, Canada

CAMILA E. ORSSO, MSc
Research Assistant, Human Nutrition Research Unit, Department of Agricultural, Food, and Nutritional Science, University of Alberta, Edmonton, Alberta, Canada

FRANCESCO COSIMO PAGANO, MD
Gemelli Against COVID-19 Post-acute Care Study Group, Fondazione Policlinico Universitario Agostino Gemelli IRCCS, Rome, Italy

CRISTINA PAIS, MD
Gemelli Against COVID-19 Post-acute Care Study Group, Geriatrician, Fondazione Policlinico Universitario Agostino Gemelli IRCCS, Rome, Italy

SIMONA PELLEGRINO, MD
Fondazione Policlinico Universitario Agostino Gemelli, IRCSS, Rome, Italy

LI-NING PENG, MD, PhD
Center for Healthy Longevity and Aging Sciences, National Yang Ming Chiao Tung University, Center for Geriatrics and Gerontology, Taipei Veterans General Hospital, Taipei, Taiwan

ERIKA PERO, MD
Fondazione Policlinico Universitario Agostino Gemelli, IRCSS, Rome, Italy

ANNA PICCA, PhD
Researcher, Center for Geriatric Medicine, Fondazione Policlinico Universitario Agostino Gemelli IRCCS, Rome, Italy

CARLA M. PRADO, PhD, RD
Professor, Human Nutrition Research Unit, Department of Agricultural, Food, and Nutritional Science, University of Alberta, Edmonton, Alberta, Canada

FRANCESCA REMELLI, MD
PhD Student, Department of Medical Science, University of Ferrara, Ferrara, Italy

SARA ROCCHI, MD
Gemelli Against COVID-19 Post-acute Care Study Group, Fondazione Policlinico Universitario Agostino Gemelli IRCCS, Rome, Italy

LEOCADIO RODRIGUEZ-MAÑAS, PhD, MD
Geriatrician, Head of Department, Servicio de Geriatría, Hospital Universitario de Getafe, Centro de Investigación Biomédica en Red "Fragilidad y Envejecimiento Saludable" (CIBERFES), Instituto de Salud Carlos III, Madrid, Spain

ISABEL RODRIGUEZ-SANCHEZ, PhD, MD
Geriatrician, Geriatrics Department, Hospital Clínico San Carlos, Madrid, Spain

YVES ROLLAND, MD, PhD
Gerontopole of Toulouse, Institute on Aging, Toulouse University Hospital (CHU Toulouse), CERPOP Centre d'Epidémiologie et de Recherche en santé des POPulations UPS/INSERM UMR 1295, Toulouse, France

ELISABETTA ROTA, MD
Gemelli Against COVID-19 Post-acute Care Study Group, Fondazione Policlinico Universitario Agostino Gemelli IRCCS, Rome, Italy

CATHERINE M. SAID, B App Sci (Physio), PhD
Department of Physiotherapy, The University of Melbourne, Melbourne, Victoria, Australia; Department of Physiotherapy, Western Health, Australia; Australian Institute for Musculoskeletal Science (AIMSS), The University of Melbourne and Western Health, St Albans, Victoria, Australia

PASCAL SAIDLITZ, MD
Gerontopole of Toulouse, Institute on Aging, Toulouse University Hospital (CHU Toulouse), Toulouse, France

ANDREA SALERNO, MD
Gemelli Against COVID-19 Post-acute Care Study Group, Fondazione Policlinico Universitario Agostino Gemelli IRCCS, Rome, Italy

GABRIELE SANI, MD
Gemelli Against COVID-19 Post-acute Care Study Group, Fondazione Policlinico Universitario Agostino Gemelli IRCCS, Rome, Italy

GIULIA SAVERA, MSc
Dietician, Fondazione Policlinico Universitario Agostino Gemelli IRCCS, Rome, Italy

MARIA EUGENIA SOTO, MD, PhD
Gerontopole of Toulouse, Institute on Aging, Toulouse University Hospital (CHU Toulouse), CERPOP Centre d'Epidémiologie et de Recherche en santé des POPulations UPS/INSERM UMR 1295, Toulouse, France

LEONARDO STELLA, MD
Gemelli Against COVID-19 Post-acute Care Study Group, Fondazione Policlinico Universitario Agostino Gemelli IRCCS, Rome, Italy

MATTEO TOSATO, MD, PhD
Gemelli Against COVID-19 Post-acute Care Study Group, Geriatrician, Fondazione Policlinico Universitario Agostino Gemelli IRCCS, Rome, Italy

CATERINA TREVISAN, MD, PhD
Assistant Professor, Department of Medical Science, University of Ferrara, Azienda Ospedaliero-Universitaria Sant'Anna, Ferrara, Italy

MARCELLO TRITTO, MD
Gemelli Against COVID-19 Post-acute Care Study Group, Fondazione Policlinico Universitario Agostino Gemelli IRCCS, Rome, Italy

STEFANO VOLPATO, MD, MPH
Full Professor of Geriatrics, Department of Medical Science, University of Ferrara, Azienda Ospedaliero-Universitaria Sant'Anna, Ferrara, Italy

MARIA BEATRICE ZAZZARA, MD
Geriatrician, Center for Geriatric Medicine, Fondazione Policlinico Universitario Agostino Gemelli IRCCS, Rome, Italy

Contents

> COVID-19 pandemic forced countries to adopt strategies aimed at responding to the health emergency by containing contagion. Lockdowns have ensured the achievement of this goal but imposed substantial restrictions to the freedom of movement and resulted in social isolation for a large share of vulnerable people. The aim of the present study was to evaluate the impact of COVID-19 pandemic and associated emergency restriction measures on the quality of life, lifestyle habits, and psychosocial status in older adults.

> Aging has been identified as one of the most relevant risk factors for poor outcomes in COVID-19 infection. Since now, different mechanisms responsible for worse outcomes in the elderly have been proposed, which include the remodeling of immune system, the higher prevalence of malnutrition and sarcopenia, the increased burden of multimorbidity, and, to a lesser extent, the direct effects of age on the respiratory system and hormonal profile. It seems that the interplay between all these causes, rather than the individual pathophysiological mechanism, explains the increased severity of the disease with age.

> Severe coronavirus disease 2019 (COVID-19) is associated with overproduction of proinflammatory cytokines. The ensuing cytokine storm contributes to the development of severe pneumonia and, possibly, to long-term symptom persistence (long COVID). The chronic state of low-grade inflammation that accompanies aging (inflammaging) might predispose older adults to severe COVID-19. Inflammaging may also contribute to symptom persistence following acute COVID-19. Antiinflammatory drugs and immunomodulatory agents can achieve significant therapeutic gain during acute COVID-19. Lifestyle interventions (eg, physical activity, diet) may be

proposed as strategies to counteract inflammation and mitigate long-term symptom persistence.

Covid-19 clinical presentation is extremely heterogenous, especially in older patients due to the possible presence of atypical symptoms, such as delirium, hyporexia and falls. The clinical characteristics at onset are influenced by the presence of common health-related conditions in older people, such as comorbidity, disability and frailty, and not simply by chronological age. Few studies investigated the tendency of Covid-19 symptoms to aggregate in cluster and the use of cluster approach might better describe the clinical complexity of the acute disease. Concerning the prognostic significance of Covid-19 clinical presentation in older people, the available literature still provides discordant results.

Patients with cognitive impairment have paid a heavy price for the coronavirus disease 2019 pandemic. Their clinical characteristics and their place of life made them particularly exposed to being infected and suffering from severe forms. The repercussions of the isolation measures also had significant repercussions on the expression of their neuropsychiatric symptoms and the burden on families and health care professionals.

It is now more than 2 years since the beginning of the COVID-19 pandemic, which has affected people around the globe, particularly older persons, who are at the highest risk of severe disease. In addition, many of those who survive will have symptoms that persist after the initial infection. COVID-19 infection severely affects function and mobility through its impact on the musculoskeletal system. This article focuses on the impact of the COVID-19 pandemic on physical activity in older people and subsequent effects and implications for function and quality of life.

Long coronavirus disease 2019 (COVID-19) is characterized by persistent COVID-19 symptoms that last for at least 2 months. In the elderly population, apart from the typical symptoms (fatigue, cough, or dyspnea), unspecific symptoms coexist (functional deterioration, cognitive impairment, or delirium) that can mitigate the prevalence of this syndrome in this age group. Its main consequence is the functional decline, leading to sarcopenia, frailty, and disability, in addition to the nutritional and cognitive disorders. Thus, a multicomponent and individualized program (exercise, diet, cognitive stimulation) should be designed for older people with persistent COVID, where new technologies could be useful.

COVID-19 negatively impacts several organs and systems weeks or months after initial diagnosis. Skeletal muscle can be affected, leading to fatigue, lower mobility, weakness, and poor physical performance. Older adults are at increased risk of developing musculoskeletal symptoms during long COVID. Systemic inflammation, physical inactivity, and poor nutritional status are some of the mechanisms leading to muscle dysfunction in individuals with long COVID. Current evidence suggests that long COVID negatively impacts body composition, muscle function, and quality of life. Muscle mass and function assessments can contribute toward the identification, diagnosis, and management of poor muscle health resulting from long COVID.

Malnutrition has been one of the most common complications of older COVID-19 survivors. COVID-19 associated symptoms like loss of appetite as well as changes in taste and smell may trigger the deterioration of nutritional status, while other complications of the disease may contribute to it, like respiratory failure that necessitates admission to the ICU. Especially in nursing home residents reduced food intake may be related to preexisting and also to incident geriatric syndromes like delirium. Sarcopenia has also been highly prevalent in older COVID-19 survivors. It is caused and exacerbated by COVID-19-associated inflammatory processes, total or partial immobilization, and malnutrition. COVID-19 survivors may be at high risk of developing the vicious circle that results from the interaction of deteriorating nutritional status and declining functionality. Regular monitoring of nutritional and functional status is, therefore, indicated in all older COVID-19 survivors. If malnutrition and/or functional decline have been identified in this patient population, low-threshold provision of individualized nutritional and exercise interventions should be installed. In those that are most seriously affected by malnutrition and sarcopenia ambulatory or inpatient rehabilitation has to be considered. Geriatric rehabilitation programs should be specifically adapted to the needs of older patients with COVID-19.

The persistence of COVID-19 symptoms weeks or months after an initial SARS-CoV-2 infection has become one of the most burdensome legacies of the pandemic. This condition, known as long COVID syndrome, affects many persons of all age groups and is associated with substantial reductions of quality of life. Several mechanisms may be involved in long COVID syndrome, including chronic inflammation, metabolic perturbations, endothelial dysfunction, and gut dysbiosis. These pathogenic mechanisms overlap with those of the aging process and may aggravate pre-existing degenerative conditions. This review discusses bioactive foods, supplements, and nutraceuticals as possible interventions against long COVID syndrome.

Alessandra Lauria, Angelo Carfi, Francesca Benvenuto, Giulia Bramato, Francesca Ciciarello, Sara Rocchi, Elisabetta Rota, Andrea Salerno, Leonardo Stella, Marcello Tritto, Antonella Di Paola, Cristina Pais, Matteo Tosato, Delfina Janiri, Gabriele Sani, Francesco Cosimo Pagano, Massimo Fantoni, Roberto Bernabei, Francesco Landi, and Alessandra Bizzarro on behalf of Gemelli Against COVID-19 Post-Acute Care Team

Coronavirus disease 2019 is known to impact older people more severely and to cause persistent symptoms during the recovery phase, including cognitive and neurologic ones. We investigated the cognitive and neurologic features of 100 elderly patients with confirmed diagnosis of coronavirus disease 2019 evaluated in the postacute phase through a direct neuropsychological evaluation consisting on Mini Mental State Examination and 8 neuropsychological tests. Overall, a total of 33 participants were found to perform at a level considered to be pathologic; more specifically, 33%, 23%, and 20% failed on Trial Making, Digit Span Backwards, and Frontal Evaluation Battery tests, respectively.

Chih-Kuang Liang, Wei-Ju Lee, Li-Ning Peng, Lin-Chieh Meng, Fei-Yuan Hsiao, and Liang-Kung Chen

The coronavirus disease 2019 (COVID-19) pandemic has had strong adverse impacts on vulnerable populations, such as frail older adults. The success of COVID-19 vaccine development, together with extensive global public health efforts, has brought hope to the control of the COVID-19 pandemic. Nevertheless, challenges in COVID-19 vaccine development and vaccination strategies among older people remain. This article reviews vaccinations in older adults, compares COVID-19 vaccine platforms, the efficacy and safety of COVID-19 vaccines in frail older people in long-term care settings, and the challenges of COVID-19 vaccine development and policy making for vaccination strategies in older adults.

CLINICS IN GERIATRIC MEDICINE

SERIES OF RELATED INTEREST

Primary Care: Clinics in Office Practice
https://www.primarycare.theclinics.com/
Immunology and Allergy Clinics
http://www.immunology.theclinics.com/

Preface

COVID-19 in the Geriatric Patient

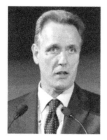

Francesco Landi, MD, PhD
Editor

After 2 years of the COVID-19 pandemic and after 1 year of vaccination campaign (with great social and economic inequality), the SARS-CoV-2 infection continues to spread quickly in many countries around the world, with the consequent respiratory illness, and still generates a very high number of affected patients and a significantly high mortality rate.[1] In this situation, the attention of researchers is mostly directed to the impact of age and multimorbidity on the prognosis of the frail and older patients. However, it became clearly evident that age and comorbidity per se are correlated with adverse outcomes but cannot systematically predict them if not associated with other conditions.

This issue addresses all the main important problems of COVID-19 in older people, from the acute phase to the chronic phase (long COVID-19), from the biological mechanisms to clinical manifestations, and also provides indications for the best care and treatment with a specific multidisciplinary approach.

During these 2 years of the COVID-19 pandemic, clinicians and pathologists have spent efforts to better characterize the site(s), nature, and severity of damage caused by SARS-CoV-2. Although the lung is definitely the first target organ of SARS-CoV-2 infection, accumulating evidence suggests that the virus can spread in many different organs, including heart, blood vessels, kidneys, gut, muscle, and brain.[2] For this reason, it is clear enough that a multidisciplinary approach becomes crucial for the evaluation and the follow-up of patients, especially older subjects, with COVID-19 disease (**Fig. 1**).

The geriatrician is the specialist who best can manage the multidimensional health problems of older subjects, with a great aptitude and skill to cope with multimorbidity and complex patients.[2] In particular, the geriatrician will be able to manage the onset of the most important geriatric syndromes, such as bed rest, sarcopenia, malnutrition, urinary incontinence, and delirium. For example, in COVID-19, nutritional status is an important factor across all disease stages from the acute to the chronic phase,[3]

Clin Geriatr Med 38 (2022) xv–xvii
https://doi.org/10.1016/j.cger.2022.05.001
0749-0690/22/© 2022 Published by Elsevier Inc.

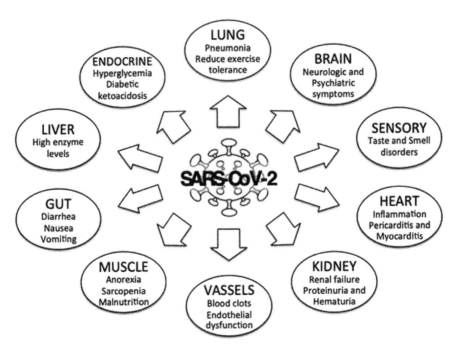

Fig. 1. Pulmonary and extrapulmonary manifestations of SARS-CoV-2 infection.

particularly in a subject at higher risk for negative outcomes, such as older frail adults and those with multimorbidities. It is widely acknowledged that malnutrition is both a cause and a consequence of immune dysfunction. In addition, in older patients with COVID-19, low levels of circulating markers of nutritional status (eg, albumin, prealbumin, lymphocyte counts) are associated with worse outcomes.[4] Prolonged in-hospital stay, especially in the intensive care unit, is a well-established risk factor for malnutrition, and leads to significant decline in muscle mass and strength and overall physical performance. It is clearly described that following SARS-CoV-2 infection, intense inflammation may aggravate catabolic processes. These phenomena may worsen malnutrition and at the same time are correlated with longest recovery, impaired physical performance, and reduced quality of life after hospital stay.[5]

Finally, the complexity of patient follow-up, the different medical specialties involved, and the possibility that some patients may develop long-term symptoms call for a multidomain organization to adequately match the needs of COVID-19 survivors. The rapid spread of the SARS-CoV-2 infection pandemic has led to an extraordinary amount of observational and experimental data focusing mainly on the acute phase of the disease. On the contrary, evidence of COVID-19 clinical history following the acute phase is quite limited, and the evidence about the long-term outcomes is not conclusive. As a consequence, it is of extreme importance that health care services organize services to ensure a comprehensive follow-up of frail older subjects suffering from the SARS-CoV-2 infection. Patient follow-up will offer an important opportunity to accumulate data in a standardized way to better define the global impact of a new disease, namely COVID-19, to better identify the specific clinical needs, and to develop comprehensive and individualized care plans for these frail patients. From this perspective, the scientific evidence reported in the articles that make up this issue is of great importance for clinicians but also for those in charge of the health care organization.

Finally, I would like to share with the readers the Gemelli Against COVID-19 Post-Acute Care (GAC19-PAC) project, the initiative developed by the Department of Geriatrics, Neuroscience and Orthopedics of the Catholic University of the Sacred Heart (Rome, Italy) aiming to respond to the needs of COVID-19 survival. With this project, the Fondazione Policlinico Universitario A. Gemelli IRCSS has set up a multi-disciplinary health care service called "Day Hospital Post-COVID-19" for all the patients recovering from the SARS-CoV-2 infection.[6]

ACKNOWLEDGMENTS

The study was supported by Ministero della Salute - Ricerca Corrente 2022.

Francesco Landi, MD, PhD
Fondazione Policlinico Universitario
"Agostino Gemelli" IRCCS
Catholic University of the Sacred Heart
L.go F. Vito 8
Rome 00168, Italy

E-mail address:
Francesco.landi@unicatt.it

REFERENCES

1. Salini S, Russo A, De Matteis G, et al. Frailty in elderly patients with Covid-19: a narrative review. Gerontol Geriatr Med 2022;8. 23337214221079956.
2. Landi F, Barillaro C, Bellieni A, et al. The new challenge of geriatrics: saving frail older people from the SARS-COV-2 pandemic infection. J Nutr Health Aging 2020;24:466–70.
3. Carfì A, Bernabei R, Landi F. Persistent symptoms in patients after acute COVID-19. JAMA 2020;32:603–5.
4. Tosato M, Carfì A, Martis I, et al. Prevalence and predictors of persistence of COVID-19 symptoms in older adults: a single-center study. J Am Med Dir Assoc 2021;22:1840–4.
5. Janiri D, Carfì A, Kotzalidis GD, et al. Post-traumatic stress disorder in patient after severe COVID-19 infection. JAMA Psychiatry 2021;78:567–9.
6. Gemelli Against COVID-19 Post-Acute Care Study Group. Post-COVID-19 global health strategies: the need for an interdisciplinary approach. Aging Clin Exp Res 2020;32:1613–20.

Lifestyle Changes and Psychological Well-Being in Older Adults During COVID-19 Pandemic

Matteo Tosato, MD, PhD[a],*, Francesca Ciciarello, MD[a],
Maria Beatrice Zazzara, MD[a], Delfina Janiri, MD[a],
Cristina Pais, MD[a], Stefano Cacciatore, MD[a],
Rossella Montenero, MD[a], Maria Sandrina Leone, MD[a],
Enea Chisci, MD[a], Anna Picca, PhD[a], Vincenzo Galluzzo, MD[a],
Hélio José Coelho-Junior, PhD[b], Riccardo Calvani, PhD[a],
Emanuele Marzetti, MD, PhD[a,b], Francesco Landi, MD, PhD[a,b], on
behalf of Gemelli Against COVID-19 Post-Acute Care Team

KEYWORDS

- Older adults • COVID-19 • Frailty • Quality of life • Mobility disorders

KEY POINTS

- Emergency restrictions aimed at reducing contagion elicited lifestyle modification.
- The impact of nonpharmacologic interventions against COVID-19 pandemic was particularly significant in older adults.
- Main consequences of restrictions in older persons were lifestyle modifications, reduced quality of life, and overall well-being, worsening in mobility and depression.

INTRODUCTION

The advent of the COVID-19 pandemic disrupted our habits and lives. The updated numbers of infections and deaths in the world's population are staggering. To date, pandemic figures reached more than 500 million cases and more than 6,000,000 deaths.[1] The risk factors for developing more severe forms of the disease are advanced age, obesity, multimorbidity, immunodeficiency, and preexisting disorders affecting lung, heart, liver, and the kidneys.[2] In particular, advanced age (85+ years) is

This study was supported by Ministero della Salute - Ricerca Corrente 2022.
[a] Fondazione Policlinico Universitario "Agostino Gemelli" IRCCS, L.go A. Gemelli 8, Rome 00168, Italy; [b] Department of Geriatrics and Orthopedics, Università Cattolica del Sacro Cuore, L.go F. Vito 8, Rome 00168, Italy
* Corresponding author.
E-mail address: matteo.tosato@policlinicogemelli.it

the most significant independent risk factor associated with intensive care unit admission and in-hospital mortality.[3]

National health systems, even those of the most developed countries, were severely challenged by COVID-19 pandemic and urged emergency political decisions aimed at containing contagion and its burdensome consequences. Large-scale nonpharmaceutical interventions were put in place, including social distancing, school closures, isolation of symptomatic people and their contacts, and generalized lockdowns.[4] Restrictive measures had a large effect in reducing SARS-CoV-2 transmission but, at the same time, heavily affected the daily life of a large share of people, including more vulnerable people.[5] Older adults, especially when multimorbid and frail, were asked to comply even more strictly with those restrictions. Despite the fact that public health measures protected thousands of older adults from the negative COVID-19 health outcomes, unintended detrimental consequences were experienced by the older age classes.[6] Notably, social isolation and reduced physical activity are well-acknowledged risk factors for negative health outcomes in the elderly population. Specifically, social isolation is associated with reduced quality of life, reduced muscle mass, cognitive function, multimorbidity, and disability.[7–9] Physical inactivity has a significant impact on health, quality of life, cognitive impairment, falls, depression, disability, hospitalization, and mortality.[10]

Moreover, study coming from previous coronavirus pandemics demonstrated impaired quality of life, depression, and psychological discomfort.[11]

In light of this evidence, several concerns exist regarding the long-term outcomes of restrictions placed on the elderly population. The aim of this study was to evaluate the impact of public health measures to mitigate COVID-19 pandemic on subjects older than 80 years, who have not suffered COVID-19, in terms of quality of life, changes in their daily habits, and psychological discomfort.

EVALUATION

We conducted an observational study in community dwellers aged 80+ years consecutively referring to the vaccination center against Sars-CoV-2 at Fondazione Policlinico Universitario Agostino Gemelli IRCCS of Rome, Italy. Participants were asked to complete a dedicated questionnaire. The questionnaire was composed of 4 sections. In the first section, demographic, anthropometric, and clinical information were collected, including age, gender, education, body height and weight, diseases, and drug therapy, together with data regarding changes in individual daily habits (such as perturbations of previous usual activities, attendance to places of worship or senior centers, physical activity routines, access to health care services). The second section evaluated the quality of life at the time of the assessment compared with the prepandemic time using a visual analogue scale (0–100). Mobility difficulty and depression status were also compared across the same timeframe. The third section assessed subjective psychological well-being using the 5-item World Health Organization Well-Being Index (WHO-5).[12,13] WHO-5 consists of 5 questions assessing the subjective well-being of the participants. The items are on a 5-point Likert scale ranging from 0 "at no time" to 5 "all of the time." The final score is calculated by summing the single items and ranges from 0 to 25, with 0 representing the worst imaginable well-being and 25 representing the best imaginable well-being. The WHO-5 is among the most widely used questionnaires assessing subjective psychological well-being, and it has showed a good internal and external validity in elderly population. A significant worsening in the quality of life was defined as a loss of at least 5 points in the visual analogue scale and/or a WHO score less than or equal to 15.

Finally, the last section assessed psychological distress related to the restrictions put in place to counteract the Sars CoV2 pandemic, through Kessler 10 Psychological Distress Scale (K10).[14] K10 is a 10-item questionnaire providing a global measure of distress based on questions about anxiety and depressive symptoms experienced in the last 4 week. Items are rated using a 5-point Likert scale ranging from 1 (never) to 5 (always). Score may range from 10 to 50. Low scores indicate low levels of psychological distress, whereas high scores indicate high levels of psychological distress. Consistently with previous validation studies[15,16] we adopted the cut-off score of greater than 19 to detect the likelihood of presence of psychological distress. The K-10 can be used with confidence in general-purpose health surveys and when assessing psychological distress in old-age communities.

At the end of the questionnaire, the study personnel assessed the frailty status of the study participants using the Clinical Frailty Status.[17]

The only exclusion criterion was the unwillingness to participate.

Statistical Analyses

Study participants were categorized into 2 groups: individuals who had changed lifestyle during the COVID-19 pandemic and individuals who reported no change. The 2 groups were compared on demographic and key clinical characteristics, quality of life, and psychological distress. Continuous variables were expressed as mean, and categorical variables were expressed as frequencies by absolute value and percentage of the total. Differences in proportions and means between the 2 groups were assessed using Fisher exact test and t-test statistics, respectively. The level of statistical significance was set at $P>.05$. Factors significantly associated with lifestyle change in bivariate analyses, together with age and sex, subsequently underwent a multivariate logistic regression to generate odds atios (ORs) and their 95% confidence intervals, with lifestyle change as dependent outcome measure. We examined possible multicollinearity between variables of interest by ensuring that the variance inflation factor indicator obtained from linear regression analysis was less than 4. We used the statistical routines of SPSS Statistics 24.0 for Windows (IBM Co., Armonk, New York, USA).

DISCUSSION

We collected data from 504 participants; main characteristics are summarized in **Table 1**. Briefly, mean age of our population was 83.2 years, and 56% were women. More common diseases were hypertension (55%), arrhythmia (16%), diabetes (15%), ischemic heart disease (11%), any cancer (10%), and osteoarthritis (10%). Mean number of diseases was 2.1 and mean number of drugs 3.6. Most of the participants had taken flu vaccination (85%), whereas only 36% had taken pneumococcal vaccination. Around 78% of participants performed routine blood check in the previous year, and 64% were visited by general practitioners. The mean score of clinical frailty scale was 3.5 ± 1.3.

We stratified our study sample into 2 groups, based on their self-reported change in daily routines. In the whole study sample, 284 older adults (56.3%) reported substantial lifestyle changes following COVID-19 pandemic and 220 individuals (43, 7%) preserved their prepandemic habitual activities. The 2 groups differed by age ($P = .02$), education ($P = .01$), and clinical frailty scale ($P<.01$). Specifically, study participants reporting lifestyle changes were younger, with higher level of education and a lower score at the clinical frailty scale. Furthermore, in the same group, a higher percentage of individuals reported a worsening in the quality of life compared with prepandemic time (**Table 2**). Multivariate logistic regression identified the worsening at the visual

Table 1
General and clinical characteristics of study population according to lifestyle change during COVID-19 pandemic era

| Characteristics | Total Sample (n = 504) | Lifestyle Change | | p |
		NO (n = 220)	YES (n = 284)	
Age (y)	83.2 ± 5.1	83.8 ± 4.5	82.8 ± 5.5	0.02
Gender				
Male	221 (44)	104 (47)	117 (41)	0.10
Female	283 (56)	116 (53)	167 (59)	
Education (y)	11.4 ± 5.3	10.7 ± 6.0	11.8 ± 4.7	0.01
Hypertension	276 (55)	117 (53)	159 (56)	0.28
Ischemic heart disease	55 (11)	26 (12)	29 (10)	0.34
Arrhythmia	80 (16)	32 (15)	48 (17)	0.27
Diabetes	75 (15)	36 (16)	39 (14)	0.24
Renal failure	14 (3)	6 (3)	8 (3)	0.58
COPD	33 (7)	18 (8)	15 (5)	0.13
Cancer	49 (10)	17 (8)	32 (11)	0.11
Osteoarthritis	41 (8)	18 (8)	23 (8)	0.55
Number of diseases	2.1 ± 1.4	2.3 ± 1.5	2.1 ± 1.2	0.12
Number of drugs	3.6 ± 2.8	3.8 ± 2.9	3.5 ± 2.6	0.20
Flu vaccination	427 (85)	189 (86)	238 (84)	0.30
Pneumococcal vaccination	183 (36)	78 (36)	105 (37)	0.39
Routine blood check	397 (78)	166 (76)	231 (81)	0.07
General practitioner visit	321 (64)	131 (60)	190 (67)	0.05
Clinical frailty scale	3.5 ± 1.3	3.7 ± 1.3	3.3 ± 1.3	<0.01

Data are given as number (percent) for gender, diseases, flu and pneumococcal vaccination, blood check, and general practitioner visit; for all the other variables, means ± SD are reported.

analogue scale as a specific risk factor for lifestyle change (OR = 2.03; $P<.001$), whereas clinical frailty score was associated with the preservation of prepandemic activities (OR = 0.78; P = .001) (**Table 3**).

In **Fig. 1** we reported the usual activities interrupted because of the pandemic. The most affected habitual routine was the visit to relatives and friends (reported by 46.5% of study participants), followed by physical activity (45.8%), participation to religious services (19.7%), cinema and theater show attendance (18.1%), shopping (12.7%), travel (7.7%), and work activities (6.1%).

As for the mobility status, the percentage of the study participants reporting no difficulty in mobility reduced from 57.4% in the prepandemic phase to 43.2%. People reporting moderate difficulty increased from 37% to 44.7%, whereas older adults reporting severe difficulty increased from 5.6% to 12.1% (**Fig. 2**).

A similar trend was observed for the depression status. Indeed, at the time of evaluation only 43.9% reported no depression compared with 76.3% in the prepandemic time, 50.3% reported moderate depression (vs 22% pre-COVID-19 time), and 5.8% reported severe depression (vs 1.7%) (**Fig. 3**).

Older adults, in particular the multimorbid and frail older population, were the most heavily affected population segment in terms of negative health outcomes and mortality during COVID-19 pandemic.[18] The latest Italian report estimated that around 85%

Table 2
Quality of life and psychological well-being of study population according to lifestyle change during COVID-19 pandemic era*

Characteristics	Total Sample (n = 504)	Lifestyle Change NO (n = 220)	Lifestyle Change YES (n = 284)	p
Self-rated health (visual analogue scale)				
VAS pre-COVID-19	76.5 ± 16.9	75.8 ± 18.3	77.0 ± 15.8	0.42
VAS COVID-19 era	69.6 ± 19.2	70.7 ± 19.8	68.7 ± 18.8	0.25
Worsened EQ-VAS	217 (43)	75 (35)	142 (65)	*<0.001*
WHO-5: The 5-item World Health Organization Well-Being Index				
WHO-5	15.8 ± 5.2	16.3 ± 5.4	15.4 ± 5.0	0.07
WHO-5 ≤15	229 (45)	87 (39)	142 (50)	*0.01*
K10 test—Kessler Psychological Distress Scale				
K10 test	16.0 ± 4.8	15.7 ± 4.9	16.2 ± 4.8	0.23
K10 test more than 19	116 (23)	46 (21)	70 (25)	0.19

Worsened quality of life: greater than 5 points lost at VAS.
WHO-5: The World Health Organisation—Five Well-Being Index (ranging from 0 to 25, with 0 representing the worst imaginable well-being and 25 representing the best imaginable well-being).
K10 test: Kessler Psychological Distress Scale (ranging from 0 to 50, with 0 representing the better result and 50 representing the worsen result).

of deaths occurred in people aged 70 years or older.[19] However, people in the oldest age groups were also the most affected by the emergency restrictive measures put in place to contain contagion due to their intrinsic vulnerability.[20] Indeed, social distancing, loneliness, and difficulty in accessing care caused by the anti-COVID-19 public health measures may have further increased the risk for several negative outcomes, including reduction of quality of life, cognitive impairment, falls, depression, disability.[21]

Studies on the topic showed conflicting results. A study conducted in individuals aged 50+ years from Italy, Spain, and France reported that about 50% of participants felt sad or depressed more often than usual during the lockdown.[22] Similarly, in Australian older adults receiving home- and community-based services, quality of life significantly worsened during the pandemic compared with the previous year.[23]

Table 3
Multivariate logistic regression (NO lifestyle change vs YES lifestyle change)

	OR [95% CI]	Wald	p
Gender	1.27 [0.87–1.86]	1.59	0.20
Age	0.98 [0.94–1.02]	0.90	0.34
Education	1.03 [0.99–1.06]	3.14	0.07
Heart failure	0.45 [0.20–1.05]	3.35	0.06
Clinical frailty scale	0.78 [0.67–0.91]	10.15	**0.001**
Worsened EQ-VAS	2.03 [1.38–3.00]	12.89	**<0.001**
WHO-5 ≤15	1.46 [0.98–2.16]	3.56	0.06

Significant results in bold.
Abbreviations: CI, confidence interval; OR, odds ratio; p, statistical significance.

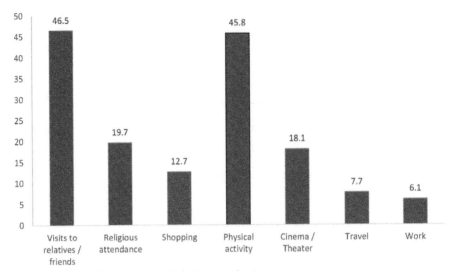

Fig. 1. Usual activities interrupted during pandemic.

In community-dwelling older adults from United States, a higher rate of depression and loneliness was reported following the onset of the pandemic.[24] In middle-aged and older adults from the Canadian Longitudinal Study on Aging the odds of depressive symptoms doubled during the pandemic compared with the prepandemic period.[25]

However, an online survey involving 825 US adults aged 60 years and older revealed that confinement/restrictions, although listed among the most stressful events of the pandemic, were not associated with negative indicators of psychological well-being.[26] Moreover, a longitudinal study conducted in Sweden concluded that COVID-19 had only minimal effects on well-being in older adults.[27] Notably, in the early pandemic phase, many Swedish older adults rated their well-being as

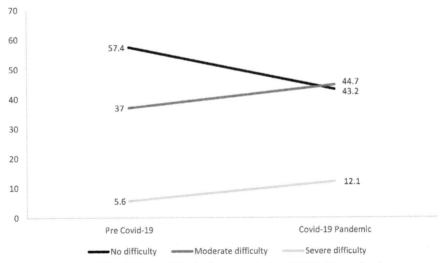

Fig. 2. Self-report difficulty in mobility before and during COVID-19 pandemic.

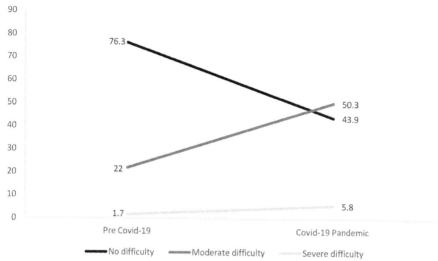

Fig. 3. Self-report depression status before and during COVID-19 pandemic.

high as or even higher than previous years. Data collected from more than 36,000 English adults of the UCL COVID-19 Social Study showed that anxiety and depressive symptoms increased during the early stages of lockdown, but with a fast improvement within a few weeks.[28]

Finally, in 720 people from the Fifth National Survey on Quality of Life in Older Adults in Chile, Herrera and colleagues found no changes in self-rated health in older adults during the pandemic, although some health indicators, including depression and anxiety, worsened.[29]

Collectively, those findings highlighted a huge heterogeneity of responses to pandemic public health measures in older adults and suggested that many older individuals may have substantial adaptive capacity and resilience.

Our results showed a significant impact of restrictive measures in community-dwelling older adults aged older than 80 years who have not contracted SARS-CoV-2 infection. Specifically, of the 504 subjects interviewed, 284 (56%) reported substantial lifestyle modifications. The main activities interrupted were visits to relatives (46%), physical activity (45.8%), attending religious services (19.7%), and cinema/theater (18.1%). Notably, although 57.4% of participants reported having no difficulty in terms of mobility before the pandemic, this percentage dropped alarmingly to 43.2%. The same pattern was observed in those who had moderate difficulty (that increased from 37% to 44.7%) and those who had severe difficulty (from 5.6% to 12.1%) increased. Mobility is critical for living independently. Older adults who lose their mobility have poorer quality of life and higher risk of several medium- to long-term negative outcomes including falls, cognitive impairment, disability, disease, hospitalization, and death.[30–32]

In this context, the increase in mobility difficulty reported by our participants is quite concerning for the overall impact this may have from both health and socioeconomic perspectives. Not surprisingly, we also found a similar trend in depression figures, with the percentage of study participants reporting no depressive symptoms that dropped from 76.3% in the pre-COVID era to 43.9%. A concomitant increase was found for moderate and severe depression.

In addition, our data showed that people who most likely made lifestyle changes were younger, with higher education status and better Clinical Frailty Scale scores. As expected, the reduction in quality of life, as well as the reduced psychosocial well-being, was more evident in subjects who modified their lifestyles.

SUMMARY

Restrictive measures aimed at containing COVID-19 pandemic had a significant impact on lifestyle habits, quality of life, psychosocial well-being, and mobility in individuals older than 80 years who have not contracted SARS-CoV-2 infection. A comprehensive multidimensional assessment should be routinely implemented to determine and manage the potential negative consequences of public health measures on overall health status and quality of life of older adults.

CLINICS CARE POINTS

- Restrictive measures to contain COVID-19 pandemic caused substantial lifestyle modifications, reduced quality of life and psychosocial well-being, and increased mobility deficits in older adults.
- People who most likely made lifestyle changes were younger, with higher education status and better Clinical Frailty Scale scores.
- The reduction in quality of life and psychosocial well-being was more evident in subjects who modified their lifestyles.
- Approaches based on multidimensional assessments should be implemented to minimize the negative health outcomes in this vulnerable population segment.

ACKNOWLEDGMENTS

The author is grateful to thank "The Gemelli Against COVID-19 Post-Acute Care Study Group".

The Gemelli Against COVID-19 Post-Acute Care Study Group is composed as follows:

Steering committee: Landi Francesco, Gremese Elisa. *Coordination*: Bernabei Roberto, Fantoni Massimo, Antonio Gasbarrini. *Field investigators*: • *Gastroenterology team:* Settanni Carlo Romano, Porcari Serena. • *Geriatric team:* Benvenuto Francesca, Bramato Giulia, Brandi Vincenzo, Carfì Angelo, Ciciarello Francesca, Lo Monaco Maria Rita, Martone Anna Maria, Marzetti Emanuele, Napolitano Carmen, Galluzzo Vincenzo, Pagano Francesco, Pais Cristina, Rocchi Sara, Rota Elisabetta, Salerno Andrea, Tosato Matteo, Tritto Marcello, Calvani Riccardo, Zazzara Maria Beatrice, Catalano Lucio, Picca Anna, Savera Giulia. • *Infectious disease team:* Cauda Roberto, Murri Rita, Cingolani Antonella, Ventura Giulio, Taddei Eleonora, Moschese Davide, Ciccullo Arturo, Fantoni Massimo. • *Internal Medicine team:* Stella Leonardo, Addolorato Giovanni, Franceschi Francesco, Mingrone Gertrude, Zocco Maria Assunta. • *Microbiology team:* Sanguinetti Maurizio, Cattani Paola, Marchetti Simona, Posteraro Brunella, Sali Michela. • *Neurology team:* Bizzarro Alessandra, Alessandra Lauria. • *Ophthalmology team:* Rizzo Stanislao, Savastano Maria Cristina, Gambini Gloria, Cozzupoli Grazia Maria, Culiersi Carola. • *Otolaryngology team:* Passali Giulio Cesare, Paludetti Gaetano, Galli Jacopo, Crudo Fabrizio, Di Cintio Giovanni, Longobardi Ylenia, Tricarico Laura, Santantonio Mariaconsiglia, Di Cesare Tiziana, Guarino Mariateresa, Corbò Marco, Settimi Stefano, Mele Dario, Brigato Francesca. •

Pediatric team: Buonsenso Danilo, Valentini Piero, Sinatti Dario, De Rose Gabriella. •
Pneumology team: Richeldi Luca, Lombardi Francesco, Calabrese Angelo, Varone
Francesco, Leone Paolo Maria, Siciliano Matteo, Corbo Giuseppe Maria, Montemurro
Giuliano, Calvello Mariarosaria, Intini Enrica, Simonetti Jacopo, Pasciuto Giuliana, Adiletta Veronica, Sofia Carmelo, Licata Maria Angela. • *Psychiatric team:* Sani Gabriele,
Delfina Janiri, Simonetti Alessio, Modica Marco, Montanari Silvia, Catinari Antonello,
Terenzi Beatrice. • *Radiology team:* Natale Luigi, Larici Anna Rita, Marano Riccardo,
Pirronti Tommaso, Infante Amato. • *Rheumatology team:* Paglionico Annamaria, Petricca Luca, Tolusso Barbara, Alivernini Stefano, Di Mario Clara. • *Vascular team:* Santoliquido Angelo, Santoro Luca, Nesci Antonio, Di Giorgio Angela, D'Alessandro
Alessia.

DISCLOSURE

No conflict of interest to disclosure.

REFERENCES

1. WHO coronavirus (COVID-19) Dashboard | WHO coronavirus (COVID-19) Dashboard with vaccination data. Available at: https://covid19.who.int/. Accessed May 2, 2022.
2. Wolff D, Nee S, Hickey NS, et al. Risk factors for Covid-19 severity and fatality: a structured literature review. Infection 2021;49(1):15–28.
3. Kim L, Garg S, O'Halloran A, et al. Risk factors for intensive care unit admission and in-hospital mortality among hospitalized adults identified through the US coronavirus disease 2019 (COVID-19)-Associated hospitalization surveillance network (COVID-NET). Clin Infect Dis 2021;72(9):E206–14.
4. Flaxman S, Mishra S, Gandy A, et al. Estimating the effects of non-pharmaceutical interventions on COVID-19 in Europe. Nature 2020;584(7820): 257–61.
5. Gashaw T, Hagos B, Sisay M. Expected impacts of COVID-19: considering resource-limited countries and vulnerable population. Front Public Health 2021; 9. https://doi.org/10.3389/FPUBH.2021.614789.
6. Falvo I, Zufferey MC, Albanese E, et al. Lived experiences of older adults during the first COVID-19 lockdown: a qualitative study. PLoS One 2021;16(6). https://doi.org/10.1371/JOURNAL.PONE.0252101.
7. Loyola WS, Camillo CA, Torres CV, et al. Effects of an exercise model based on functional circuits in an older population with different levels of social participation. Geriatr Gerontol Int 2018;18(2):216–23.
8. Douglas H, Georgiou A, Westbrook J. Social participation as an indicator of successful aging: an overview of concepts and their associations with health. Aust Health Rev 2017;41(4):455–62.
9. Lindsay Smith G, Banting L, Eime R, et al. The association between social support and physical activity in older adults: a systematic review. Int J Behav Nutr Phys Act 2017;14(1). https://doi.org/10.1186/S12966-017-0509-8.
10. Ozemek C, Lavie CJ, Rognmo Ø. Global physical activity levels - need for intervention. Prog Cardiovasc Dis 2019;62(2):102–7.
11. Lee AM, Wong JGWS, McAlonan GM, et al. Stress and psychological distress among SARS survivors 1 year after the outbreak. Can J Psychiatry 2007;52(4): 233–40.
12. Topp CW, Østergaard SD, Søndergaard S, et al. The WHO-5 Well-Being Index: a systematic review of the literature. Psychother Psychosom 2015;84(3):167–76.

13. Staehr Johansen K. The use of wellbeing measures in primary health care/The DepCare Project. World Health Organization, Regional Office for Europe: Well-Being Measures in Primary Health Care/The DepCare Project. Published online 1998:target 12, E60246.
14. Kessler RC, Andrews G, Colpe LJ, et al. Short screening scales to monitor population prevalences and trends in non-specific psychological distress. Psychol Med 2002;32(6):959–76.
15. Kessler RC, Barker PR, Colpe LJ, et al. Screening for serious mental illness in the general population. Arch Gen Psychiatry 2003;60(2):184–9.
16. Andrews G, Slade T. Interpreting scores on the Kessler psychological distress scale (K10). Aust N Z J Public Health 2001;25(6):494–7.
17. Rockwood K, Song X, MacKnight C, et al. A global clinical measure of fitness and frailty in elderly people. CMAJ 2005;173(5):489–95.
18. Variation in the COVID-19 infection-fatality ratio by age, time, and geography during the pre-vaccine era: a systematic analysis. Lancet 2022;399(10334):1469–88.
19. COVID-19 integrated surveillance: key national data. Available at: https://www.epicentro.iss.it/en/coronavirus/sars-cov-2-integrated-surveillance-data. Accessed May 2, 2022.
20. Manca R, de Marco M, Venneri A. The impact of COVID-19 infection and enforced prolonged social isolation on neuropsychiatric symptoms in older adults with and without Dementia: a review. Front Psychiatry 2020;11. https://doi.org/10.3389/FPSYT.2020.585540.
21. Cacioppo JT, Cacioppo S. Older adults reporting social isolation or loneliness show poorer cognitive function 4 years later. Evid Based Nurs 2014;17(2):59–60.
22. Arpino B, Pasqualini M, Bordone V, et al. Older people's nonphysical contacts and depression during the COVID-19 lockdown. Gerontologist 2021;61(2):176–86.
23. Siette J, Dodds L, Seaman K, et al. The impact of COVID-19 on the quality of life of older adults receiving community-based aged care. Australas J Ageing 2021;40(1):84–9.
24. Krendl AC, Perry BL. The impact of sheltering in place during the COVID-19 pandemic on older adults' social and mental well-being. J Gerontol B Psychol Sci Soc Sci 2021;76(2):E53–8.
25. Raina P, Wolfson C, Griffith L, et al. A longitudinal analysis of the impact of the COVID-19 pandemic on the mental health of middle-aged and older adults from the Canadian Longitudinal Study on Aging. Nat Aging 2021;1(12):1137–47.
26. Whitehead BR, Torossian E. Older adults' experience of the COVID-19 pandemic: a mixed-methods analysis of stresses and joys. Gerontologist 2021;61(1):36–47.
27. Kivi M, Hansson I, Bjälkebring P. Up and about: older adults' well-being during the COVID-19 pandemic in a Swedish longitudinal study. J Gerontol B Psychol Sci Soc Sci 2021;76(2):E4–9.
28. Fancourt D, Steptoe A, Bu F. Trajectories of anxiety and depressive symptoms during enforced isolation due to COVID-19 in England: a longitudinal observational study. Lancet Psychiatry 2021;8(2):141–9.
29. Herrera MS, Elgueta R, Fernández MB, et al. A longitudinal study monitoring the quality of life in a national cohort of older adults in Chile before and during the COVID-19 outbreak. BMC Geriatr 2021;21(1). https://doi.org/10.1186/S12877-021-02110-3.
30. Rasch EK, Magder L, Hochberg MC, et al. Health of community-dwelling adults with mobility limitations in the United States: incidence of secondary health conditions. Part II. Arch Phys Med Rehabil 2008;89(2):219–30.

31. Freiberger E, Sieber CC, Kob R. Mobility in older community-dwelling persons: a narrative review. Front Physiol 2020;11. https://doi.org/10.3389/FPHYS.2020.00881.
32. Jain P, Bellettiere J, Glass N, et al. The relationship of accelerometer-assessed standing time with and without ambulation and mortality: the WHI OPACH study. J Gerontol A Biol Sci Med Sci 2021;76(1):77–84.

How can Biology of Aging Explain the Severity of COVID-19 in Older Adults

Antonella Gallo, MD[a], Erika Pero, MD[a], Simona Pellegrino, MD[a],
Noemi Macerola, MD[a], Celeste Ambra Murace, MD[a],
Francesca Ibba, MD[a], Maria Chiara Agnitelli, MD[a],
Francesco Landi, MD, PhD[a,b], Massimo Montalto, MD, PhD[a,b],*

KEYWORDS

- Aging • Comorbidities • COVID-19 • Immunosenescence • Inflammaging
- Sarcopenia • Malnutrition

KEY POINTS

- Aging has been identified as one of the most relevant risk factors for poor outcomes in COVID-19 infection, representing an important predictor both for higher mortality and disease severity.
- Different mechanisms have been proposed to explain the worse outcomes in the elderly, including the remodeling of immune system, the higher prevalence of malnutrition and sarcopenia, the increased burden of multimorbidity, and, to a lesser extent, the direct effects of age on the respiratory system and hormonal profile.
- The interplay between all these causes, rather than the individual pathophysiological mechanism, explains the increased severity of the disease with age.

Funding: none.
Author contributions: all authors contributed to the study conception and design. Material preparation, data collection, and analysis were performed by Antonella Gallo, Erika Pero, Simona Pellegrino, Noemi Macerola, Celeste Ambra Murace Francesca Ibba, and Maria Chiara Agnitelli. The first draft of the manuscript was written by Antonella Gallo, Erika Pero, Simona Pellegrino, and Noemi Macerola. All authors commented on previous versions of the manuscript. All authors read and approved the final manuscript.
[a] Fondazione Policlinico Universitario A. Gemelli, IRCSS, Rome, Italy; [b] Università Cattolica del Sacro Cuore, Rome, Italy
* Corresponding author. Fondazione Policlinico Universitario A. Gemelli, IRCCS, Largo A. Gemelli 1, Roma 00168, Italy.
E-mail addresses: antonella.gallo@policlinicogemelli.it (A.G.); pero.erika@gmail.com (E.P.); pellegrino.simona3@gmail.com (S.P.); noemi.macerola@gmail.com (N.M.); celeste.murace@gmail.com (C.A.M.); franci.ibba@gmail.com (F.I.); mariachiaragnitelli@icloud.com (M.C.A.); francesco.landi@policlinicogemelli.it (F.L.); massimo.montalto@unicatt.it (M.M.)

INTRODUCTION

In December 2019 a cluster of pneumonia caused by a previous unknown coronavirus, SARS-CoV-2, was identified in Wuhan, China.[1] SARS-CoV-2 belongs to the subgenus of beta-coronavirus,[2] as SARS-CoV and MERS-CoV, respectively emerged as epidemic in 2003 and 2012. The person-to-person transmission occurring via respiratory droplets or aerosols[3] led to a rapid spreading of COVID-19 infection,[4] firstly through China and then through all the other countries of the world, thus becoming a pandemic.[4] COVID-19 shows a high variability of clinical pictures, ranging from mild or no pneumonia (81% of cases) to severe pneumonia (14% of cases) and critical pneumonia (5% of cases).[5,6]

Aging has been identified as one of the most relevant risk factors for poor outcomes in COVID-19 disease, independently from the presence of preexisting diseases.[7,8] The COVID-19 mortality risk sharply increases for elderly subjects, as showed by the reports of China, Italy, and the United States.[7] In particular, in Italy, case fatality rate for patient aged 40 to 49 years or younger was reported of about 0.4% or lower, 1% among those aged 50 to 59 years, 3.5% in those aged 60 to 69 years, 12.8% in those aged 70 to 79 years, to 20.2% from 80 years and older.[8]

Age is not only an important predictor for mortality, but it is also associated with higher disease severity, in terms of increased hospitalization rates, length of hospital stay, need for intensive care, and invasive mechanical ventilation.[8–11] Since now, different mechanisms responsible for worse outcomes in the elderly have been suggested,[12–14] which include the remodeling of immune system, the higher prevalence of malnutrition and sarcopenia, the increased burden of multimorbidity, and, to a lesser extent, the direct effects of age on the respiratory system and hormonal profile. The interplay between all these causes, rather than the individual pathophysiological mechanism, explains the increased severity of the disease with age.[8–14]

REMODELING OF IMMUNE SYSTEM

The terms "immunosenescence" and "inflammaging" refer to age-related physiologic changes in both innate and adaptive immune system, which lead to a higher incidence of infection, cancer, and autoimmune disease in the elderly population.[15]

The decline of the immune system with age, consisting of inappropriately amplified and dysregulated immune responses,[15] leads not only to a greater susceptibility to bacterial and viral infections but also to more severe consequences of infectious disease, such as severe respiratory failure in COVID-19 infection and lowered responses to vaccination.[15,16] Interestingly, age-related remodeling of the immune system is associated with a sort of paradox: a state of increased autoimmunity and inflammation coexistent with a state of immunodeficiency.[16]

"Immunosenescence" represents the gradual deterioration of the host's ability to mount an effective immune response against new antigens, whereas "inflammaging" identifies a state of chronic, sterile low-grade inflammation resulting from the long-term physiologic stimulation of an overactive, yet ineffective, immune system. Together, these 2 mechanisms might facilitate the development of cytokine storm in elderly.[16]

Immunosenescence and COVID-19 Infection

Aging strongly affects the immune system, influencing both the humoral and cellular arm of immunity, from hematopoietic stem cells to mature lymphocytes in secondary lymphoid organs.

Since now, several hallmarks of immunosenescence have been identified. One of the salient features of this mechanism is the decrease in peripheral naïve T cell,[17,18] as a result of the fibroadipose involution of the thymus and the reduced ability of lymph nodes to store, maintain, and support naïve T cells with age. Although there is a 95% reduction in the number of naive T lymphocytes in the elderly compared with young people,[19] there is only a slight reduction in the total number of T lymphocytes in advanced age[19,20] due to the compensatory accumulation of memory T cells.[19] These senescent cells are mainly characterized by a decrease in T-cell receptor (TCR) repertoire[21] and by a reduction in the expression of the costimulatory surface protein CD28+, which is the signature of replicative senescence.[22] Indeed, CD28 is not only important in lymphocyte activation but also plays a role in telomere homeostasis.[23] Memory cells are characterized by low telomerase activity, high production of reactive oxygen species and constitutive activation of p38 mitogen-activated protein kinase, which once activated, blocks signaling via TCRs.[24] All these changes contribute to the decreased ability of the aging immune system to mount an adaptive response against new antigens.

"Immunosenescence" is also characterized by the imbalance of the Th1/Th2 ratio.[25] The host's ability to balance the differentiation of CD4 lymphocytes into Th1 phenotypes, which has a proinflammatory role, and Th2, which has an antiinflammatory function, is vital for the neutralization of pathogens without inducing damages to host tissues.[25,26] It seems that in elderly patient there is an impairment in this mechanism that would favor the development of more severe forms of COVID-19 disease.[25] Indeed, in early stage of the infection there is a predominant Th2 response that would aid viral replication, followed by a rapid upregulation of Th1 response that would lead to cytokine storm and development of critical illness.[25,27] On the same note, in the elderly population there is an upregulation of the proinflammatory pathways mediated by Th17 cells and a loss of the antiinflammatory response mediated by regulatory T cell lymphocytes.[28]

Moreover, a reduction in CD8+ T cells has also been described in severe cases of COVID-19,[29] suggesting an impairment of the host's ability to fight viruses. The functional exhaustion of the cytotoxic function of CD8+ due to the reduction of the coexpression of perforin and granzyme B,[30] has already been associated not only with an increased risk of contracting influenza infection but also with increased disease severity in elderly.[31,32]

As regarding humoral immunity, older people showed both a decrease in bone marrow output of naïve B-lymphocytes[33] and the accumulation of the double-negative B cells subtype, which are exhausted cells with functional impairment.[34,35] The accumulation of these dysfunctional B cells has been reported in healthy elderly subjects and recently in severe cases of COVID-19 disease.[36]

As a result of the decline of both T and B lymphocytes, aged individuals are characterized by an ineffective antibody response, in terms of decreased affinity, poor neutralization of antigens, and production of antibodies more prone to autoreactivity.[35] Moreover, for the same reasons, the duration of protection of immunity following vaccination is usually shortened in this population.[37]

Finally, the mechanism related to the "antibody-dependent enhancement (ADE)" has also been associated with severity of COVID-19 infection.[38] ADE is a phenomenon whereby the binding of virus to nonneutralizing antibodies, produced during other infections, promotes its internalization into host cells and facilitates the downstream inflammatory responses.[39] This mechanism has been described for other coronavirus infections, such as SARS-CoV-1 and MERS,[40,41] as well as for other viral infections (ie, dengue fever and human immunodeficiency virus).[39] It has been suggested that elderly might be more prone to these mechanism because of the exposition of a lifetime to circulating virus.[13]

Inflammaging and COVID-19 Infection

Older patients may show a baseline low-grade inflammation in the absence of infectious processes.[42] This condition, called "inflammaging", is characterized by high baseline serum concentration of C-reactive protein and cytokines (interleukin-6 [IL-6] and IL-8) and is associated with increased fragility and morbidity.[42] Inflammaging may be the result of multiple mechanisms, including the accumulation of misfolded proteins, the gut barrier leaking, and obesity.[43] Moreover, elderly may be characterized by an impaired clearance of dead and dying cells from sites of immune activity,[42] leading to persistent inflammation, and by the presence of senescent cells, which do not proliferate but secrete inflammatory molecules (process known as the senescence-associated secretory phenotype).[22] This excessive inflammation can negatively affect some functions of the immune system.[42] It has been suggested that in COVID-19 lung infections, the presence of a preexisting inflammatory condition and senescent cells can lead to the development of an exacerbated cytokine storm, with recruitment of other inflammatory cells.[42] Molecules such as tumor necrosis factor alpha (TNF-α), IL-6, IL-1β, and monocyte chemoattractant protein-1 determine the expression of natural killer cell receptor (NKR) ligand by nonlymphoid cells of the respiratory tract and lungs, which can be targeted and killed by infiltrating aged T cells expressing NKRs, causing tissue and organ damage.[42]

Severity of COVID-19 disease has also been correlated to the neutrophil-lymphocyte ratio, which usually indicates low-grade inflammation in elderly, as in obesity, metabolic syndrome, and diabetes.[44]

COMORBIDITIES

Several epidemiologic studies reported that the presence of preexisting comorbidities represents a relevant risk factor in patients with COVID-19 for a more severe disease in terms of increased and prolonged hospitalizations and mortality.[45–51]

The most common comorbidities found in cohorts of patients with COVID-19 were diabetes, hypertension, obesity, chronic cardiovascular, pulmonary, and kidney diseases.[45–52] These are all medical conditions characterized by a state of chronic inflammation associated with a weakened immune response that could explain the predisposition to infections and disease complications.

Although there are many studies investigating the role of comorbidities in COVID-19 disease in the general population, there are not many data addressing the association between comorbidities and aging. A Spanish retrospective study including 834 patients aged 60 years and older, hospitalized for COVID-19, showed that patients with heart failure and chronic kidney disease had an increased risk of hospital mortality.[52] A retrospective study conducted on 889 patients showed that the presence of multimorbidity, identified by an increased Charlson Comorbidity Index, together with the presence of symptoms and advanced age (>60 years), was associated with an increase in hospitalization, severity, and fatality in patients with COVID-19.[53]

When stratifying impact of comorbidities in different age subgroups (<50 years, 50–69 years, and 70–90 years), Harrison and colleagues showed that in a total of 31,461 patients with COVID-19, history of myocardial infarction or chronic kidney disease was associated with higher risk of mortality for all groups.[54] Instead, significant differences were found across age subgroups for other chronic conditions and their association with mortality. In particular, in subjects aged 70 to 90 years, congestive heart failure and dementia were significantly associated with higher risk of mortality.[54]

Relevant data on impact of comorbidities in older patients with COVID-19 are also derived from studies on skilled nursing facilities where, mainly during the first outbreak, a rapid virus transmission between residents was reported.[55] In a context of a US nursing facility, during the rapidly escalating COVID-19 outbreak in March 2020, McMichael and colleagues found a death percentage of 33.7% for residents, in respect to 6.2% for visitors and 0% for staff. Residents showed a medium age of 83 years, most of them having one or more comorbidities, such as hypertension (67%), chronic cardiac disease (60%), kidney disease (41%), diabetes (32%).[55]

The postulated mechanisms for a worse prognosis in these comorbid and older patients mainly include the dysregulation of the immune system associated with chronic low-grade inflammation favoring cytokine storm, the prothrombotic state and endothelial dysfunction with consequent increased risk of thromboembolic events, and the dysregulated and widespread angiotensin enzyme 2 (ACE2) activity promoting viral uptake, as better described in the following paragraphs.

Diabetes represents one of the commonest comorbidities, whose prevalence in patients with COVID-19 ranges from 7.3% in China[5] to more than 30% in Europe.[56] Diabetes does not seem to increase the incidence of SARS-CoV-2 infection,[57,58] but it can unfavorably modify the course of the disease, with an increased risk of disease progression, with development of acute respiratory distress syndrome and multiorgan failure and higher mortality rate.[59] Moreover, retrospective studies showed that patients with COVID-19 diabetes had higher levels of inflammatory biomarkers (such as neutrophil-to-lymphocyte ratio, high-sensitivity C-reactive protein, and procalcitonin) when compared with nondiabetes patients.[60–62] Therefore, diabetes has been recognized as an independent risk factor for poor prognosis in patients with COVID-19. However, when stratifying diabetic subjects to identify those at higher risk of death, Schlesinger and colleagues showed in their meta-analysis that older age (>65 years) was significantly associated with higher risk of COVID-19–associated death and with COVID-19 severity.[63] Reasons for higher COVID-19 complications in this subgroup of diabetics were mainly related to glycemic instability and association with preexiting comorbidities, such as hypertension, cardiovascular, and kidney disease, together with the suggested influence of a chronic low-grade inflammation and factors associated with viral entry (such as ACE2 expression).[60–63]

SARCOPENIA AND MALNUTRITION IN COVID-19 INFECTION

A sufficient protein intake and a good nutritional status are required for an optimal antibody production and for the synthesis of acute-phase proteins (C-reactive protein, ferritin, interleukins, TNF-α).[64] Therefore, an inadequate protein intake or vitamin and trace element deficiencies can lead to weakened immune responses. The risk of malnutrition in geriatric patients is increased compared with the general population. "Anorexia of aging" is a disorder characterized by a reduction of food intake and/or loss of appetite in elderly patients, and it is an independent predictor of worse prognosis.[65] Some physiologic age-related factors are involved in the development of anorexia in elderly patients (reduction of smell and taste, changes among hunger and satiety hormones, chronic low-grade inflammation, abnormality in gastric motility), as well as social (eg, poverty, isolation), psychological (eg, depression, dementia), medical (eg, edentulism, dysphagia, malignancy), and pharmacologic factors.[65]

COVID-19 itself can be a cause of malnutrition, due to the infectious involvement of the gastrointestinal tract with consequent malabsorption.[6,64] It can be also responsible for sarcopenia, due to the acute inflammatory response or as a consequence of the treatment with glucocorticoids.[64] Damayanthi and colleagues conducted a systematic review on correlation between nutritional status of older patient and COVID-19 outcome, highlighting that the prevalence of malnutrition in these patients is high and negatively influences their prognosis.[64] In particular, Recinella and colleagues, in a cross-sectional study on 109 patients, showed that a moderate/severe geriatric nutritional risk index (GNRI) represented a risk factor for in-hospital death, whereas body mass index represented a protective factor.[66] Two other studies found that either albumin levels (by an observational longitudinal study on 114 patients)[67] or prealbumin levels (by a retrospective cohort study on 446 patients)[68] were associated with a higher risk of transfer to intensive care unit (ICU) and all cause of death, ICU admission, and mechanical ventilation, respectively.

Sarcopenia also affects the respiratory and swallowing muscles. A reduction in the respiratory muscle strength hinders effective coughing.[69] Okazaki and colleagues reported that malnutrition, lower body trunk muscle mass, and respiratory muscle weakness represent risk factors for pneumonia in elderly, and malnutrition represents a risk factor for pneumonia relapse.[69]

Considering that underweight has been correlated with a higher probability of hospitalization in adult patients with viral respiratory infections from coronavirus, metapneumovirus, parainfluenza, and rhinovirus[70] and that malnutrition in the elderly can significantly influence regulatory T cells and senescent natural killer cells, increasing the risk of infections, Lidoriki and colleagues speculated about a possible association between malnutrition in elderly people and COVID-19 prognosis.[70] In particular, they suggested that a combination of a respiratory infection severity score such as CURB-65, malnutrition (GNRI), and performance status (The Eastern Cooperative Oncology Group, Barthel) scores could represent a quick and low-cost prognostic tool for COVID-19 in the elderly.[70]

ULTRASTRUCTURAL CHANGES AND COVID-19 INFECTION

Aging is also associated with ultrastructural changes in the respiratory system, including decline in the clearance of inhaled particles at the level of small airways,[71] gradual reduction in the number of cilia and ciliated cells in the airways, impairment in nasal mucociliary clearance with a slower ciliary beat frequency,[72] and increase in nasal cavity with a decrease in nasal resistance.[73] All the aforementioned changes may contribute to the higher prevalence of respiratory infection and COVID-19 in the elderly.

ACE2 receptor represents the human door for SARS-CoV and SARS-CoV-2 entry into cells and plays a pivotal role in the pathogenesis of COVID-19 disease.[74] ACE2 receptor, a transmembrane type I glycoprotein, is not only expressed by nasal epithelium and type II alveolar cells but also in other tissues (myocardium, kidney, urothelial, ileum, colon, esophagus, and oral mucosa cells), thus explaining the systemic presentation of COVID-19 disease.[75] In human physiology, soluble ACE2 cleaves angiotensin II to angiotensin, limiting the detrimental effects of angiotensin II receptor type I receptors, including vasoconstriction, inflammation, and thrombosis.[76,77] After the binding of SARS-CoV-2 to ACE2 receptors, the spike proteins of both SARS- CoV and SARS-CoV-2 by priming a transmembrane serine protease (TMPRSS2) causes the internalization and degradation of ACE2, with downregulation of these receptors.[77,78] By this way, the decrease of ACE2 activity exacerbates the severity of lung injuries and inflammatory pulmonary diseases, mediated by angiotensin II.[78]

Several factors have been shown to affect the expression of ACE2 and consequently cause the shift of ACE/ACE2 balance toward proinflammatory and profibrotic effects mediated by ACE and the ACE-angiotensin II-AT1 receptor axis.[76,77] Aging is one of these factors. Recent evidence suggests that a decrease in the expression of ACE2 with age could lead to exaggerated inflammatory responses and cytokine storm.[79] Moreover, genomics and transcriptomics studies have shown an age-related reduction in the expression of ACE2 receptors in many tissues.[80]

Interestingly, different chronic diseases associated with COVID-19 infection and typical of older age, such as hypertension, diabetes, and cardiac disease, share a variable degree of ACE2 deficiency.[75–77] In these conditions, the consequent angiotensin II effects may result in exacerbation of hypertension, cardiac hypertrophy, and maladaptive left ventricular remodeling after a myocardial infarction.[75]

Therefore, ACE2 deficiency seems to play a key role in the pathogenesis but also in the prognosis of COVID-19 infection, mainly in those subjects (ie, elderly and with comorbidities) with baseline ACE2 deficiency.

HORMONAL CHANGES

Among the elderly population, men have a higher risk of death from COVID-19 than women.[81] The reasons for this difference are still under investigation. One of the hypotheses concerns the reduced testosterone levels in elderly men and the related consequences on general health and the immune system.[81]

In men, testosterone levels progressively decline from the age of 30 years.[81] In the elderly men, low testosterone levels can be associated with various symptoms, including loss of libido, erectile dysfunction, and loss of muscle mass, among other symptoms, as well as a greater likelihood of both metabolic syndrome and cardiovascular disease. Reduced testosterone levels and the presence of such symptoms is referred to as late-onset hypogonadism[82] and have also been associated with increased frailty[83] and mortality.[84]

In women there is a progressive reduction of testosterone levels between 20 and 40 years,[85,86] whereas between 60 and 80 years they can increase in varying degrees.[86,87] Testosterone levels in older women do not seem to play a significant role in increasing the risk of frailty.[83]

Papadopoulos and colleagues hypothesized that reduced testosterone levels in elderly men could be associated with increased COVID-19 mortality.[81] One of the reasons may be the inhibitory role of testosterone on the immune system, by reducing the expression of inflammatory mediators (eg, IL-6) and promoting antiinflammatory responses. High levels of IL-6 have been linked to the development of the acute respiratory distress syndrome (ARDS) in COVID-19 infections, and elderly male patients showed a higher risk to develop ARDS and death.[81]

It is also possible that SARS-Cov-2 can act directly on testicular function and testosterone levels. It has been shown in fact that Leydig cells express ACE2 and also TMPRSS2, leading testis to represent another potential target of SARS-CoV2.

SUMMARY

In conclusion, increasing age represents an unquestionable risk factor for poor outcomes in COVID-19 infection. Common features of older people, such as increased incidence of comorbidities, dysregulation of immune system, and malnutrition, interplay with ultrastructural changes of aged systems (mainly the respiratory one) in exacerbating inflammatory deleterious pathways triggered by SARS-CoV-2 virus. In this context, ACE2 role is deserving a lot of interest as key mechanism involved in pathogenesis and evolution of disease, although data on the older subgroups are scarce and mostly theoretic. Further and more specific studies should be encouraged to better understand all these mechanisms, in order to achieve targeted approaches and, hopefully, preventive strategies in frail subjects, such as the elderly.

CLINICS CARE POINTS

- Age represents one of the most relevant risk factor for poor outcome in the majority of diseases.
- The terms "immunosenescence" and "inflammaging" are deserving increased attention.
- However, mechanisms involved in age-related more severe course of common disease are not fully understood.

CONFLICT OF INTERESTS

All authors declare that they have no conflict of interest.

REFERENCES

1. Zhu N, Zhang D, Wang W, et al. A novel coronavirus from patients with pneumonia in China, 2019. N Engl J Med 2020;382(8):727–33.
2. Zhou P, Yang XL, Wang XG, et al. A pneumonia outbreak associated with a new coronavirus of probable bat origin. Nature 2020;579(7798):270–3.
3. Shereen MA, Khan S, Kazmi A, et al. COVID-19 infection: origin, transmission, and characteristics of human coronaviruses. J Adv Res 2020;24:91–8.
4. WHO Director-General's remarks at the media briefing on 2019-nCoV on 11 February 2020. Available at: https://www.who.int/director-general/speeches/detail/. Accessed February 11, 2020.
5. Wu Z, McGoogan JM. Characteristics of and important lessons from the Coronavirus Disease 2019 (COVID-19) outbreak in China: summary of a report of 72 314 cases from the Chinese Center for disease control and prevention. JAMA 2020;323(13):1239–42.
6. Huang C, Wang Y, Li X, et al. Clinical features of patients infected with 2019 novel coronavirus in Wuhan, China. Lancet Lond Engl 2020;395(10223):497–506.
7. Chen Y, Klein SL, Garibaldi BT, et al. Aging in COVID-19: vulnerability, immunity and intervention. Ageing Res Rev 2021;65:101205.
8. Onder G, Rezza G, Brusaferro S. Case-fatality rate and characteristics of patients dying in relation to COVID-19 in Italy. JAMA 2020;323(18):1775–6.
9. Li X, Xu S, Yu M, et al. Risk factors for severity and mortality in adult COVID-19 inpatients in Wuhan. J Allergy Clin Immunol 2020;146(1):110–8.
10. Salje H, TranKiem C, Lefrancq N, et al. Estimating the burden of SARS-CoV-2 in France. Science 2020;369(6500):208–11.
11. CDC COVID-19 Response Team. Severe outcomes among patients with Coronavirus Disease 2019 (COVID-19) - United States, February 12-March 16, 2020. MMWR Morb Mortal Wkly Rep 2020;69(12):343–6.
12. Bajaj V, Gadi N, Spihlman AP, et al. Aging, Immunity, and COVID-19: how age influences the host immune response to coronavirus infections? Front Physiol 2021;11:571416.
13. Pietrobon AJ, Teixeira FME, Sato MN. Immunosenescence and inflammaging: risk factors of severe COVID-19 in older people. Front Immunol 2020;11:579220.
14. Perrotta F, Corbi G, Mazzeo G, et al. COVID-19 and the elderly: insights into pathogenesis and clinical decision-making. Aging Clin Exp Res 2020;32(8):1599–608.
15. Fuentes E, Fuentes M, Alarcón M, et al. Immune system dysfunction in the elderly. An Acad Bras Ciênc 2017;89:285–99.

16. Sardi F, Fassina L, Venturini L, et al. Alzheimer's disease, autoimmunity and inflammation. The good, the bad and the ugly. Autoimmun Rev 2011;11(2): 149–53.
17. Linton PJ, Dorshkind K. Age-related changes in lymphocyte development and function. Nat Immunol 2004;5(2):133–9.
18. Stahl EC, Brown BN. Cell therapy strategies to combat immunosenescence. Organogenesis 2015;11(4):159–72.
19. Ponnappan S, Ponnappan U. Aging and immune function: molecular mechanisms to interventions. Antioxid Redox Signal 2011;14(8):1551–85.
20. Sprent J, Surh CD. Normal T cell homeostasis: the conversion of naive cells into memory-phenotype cells. Nat Immunol 2011;12(6):478–84.
21. Britanova OV, Putintseva EV, Shugay M, et al. Age-related decrease in TCR repertoire diversity measured with deep and normalized sequence profiling. J Immunol 2014;192(6):2689–98.
22. Vallejo AN. CD28 extinction in human T cells: altered functions and the program of T-cell senescence. Immunol Rev 2005;205:158–69.
23. Plunkett FJ, Franzese O, Finney HM, et al. The loss of telomerase activity in highly differentiated CD8+CD28−CD27− T cells is associated with decreased Akt (Ser473) Phosphorylation. J Immunol 2007;178(12):7710–9.
24. Akbar AN, Henson SM, Lanna A. Senescence of T lymphocytes: implications for enhancing human immunity. Trends Immunol 2016;37(12):866–76.
25. Ye Q, Wang B, Mao J. The pathogenesis and treatment of the Cytokine Storm' in COVID-19. J Infect 2020;80(6):607–13.
26. De Biasi S, Meschiari M, Gibellini L, et al. Marked T cell activation, senescence, exhaustion and skewing towards TH17 in patients with COVID-19 pneumonia. Nat Commun 2020;11(1):3434.
27. Har-Noy M, Or R. Allo-priming as a universal anti-viral vaccine: protecting elderly from current COVID-19 and any future unknown viral outbreak. J Transl Med 2020;18(1):196.
28. Schmitt V, Rink L, Uciechowski P. The Th17/Treg balance is disturbed during aging. Exp Gerontol 2013;48(12):1379–86.
29. Zhou Y, Fu B, Zheng X, et al. Pathogenic T-cells and inflammatory monocytes incite inflammatory storms in severe COVID-19 patients. Natl Sci Rev 2020; 7(6):998–1002.
30. Thiery J, Keefe D, Boulant S, et al. Perforin pores in the endosomal membrane trigger the release of endocytosed granzyme B into the cytosol of target cells. Nat Immunol 2011;12(8):770–7.
31. McElhaney JE, Zhou X, Talbot HK, et al. The unmet need in the elderly: how immunosenescence, CMV infection, co-morbidities and frailty are a challenge for the development of more effective influenza vaccines. Vaccine 2012;30(12): 2060–7.
32. Shahid Z, Kleppinger A, Gentleman B, et al. Clinical and immunologic predictors of influenza illness among vaccinated older adults. Vaccine 2010;28(38): 6145–51.
33. Chinn IK, Blackburn CC, Manley NR, et al. Changes in primary lymphoid organs with aging. Semin Immunol 2012;24(5):309–20.
34. Frasca D, Diaz A, Romero M, et al. Human peripheral late/exhausted memory B cells express a senescent-associated secretory phenotype and preferentially utilize metabolic signaling pathways. Exp Gerontol 2017;87(Pt A):113–20.
35. Frasca D, Diaz A, Romero M, et al. B cell immunosenescence. Annu Rev Cell Dev Biol 2020;36:551–74.

36. Woodruff MC, Ramonell RP, Nguyen DC, et al. Extrafollicular B cell responses correlate with neutralizing antibodies and morbidity in COVID-19. Nat Immunol 2020;21(12):1506–16.
37. Crooke SN, Ovsyannikova IG, Poland GA, et al. Immunosenescence and human vaccine immune responses. Immun Ageing A 2019;16:25.
38. Peron JPS, Nakaya H. Susceptibility of the elderly to SARS-CoV-2 infection: ACE-2 overexpression, shedding, and antibody-dependent enhancement (ADE). Clin Sao Paulo Braz 2020;75:e1912.
39. Tirado SMC, Yoon KJ. Antibody-dependent enhancement of virus infection and disease. Viral Immunol 2003;16(1):69–86.
40. Tetro JA. Is COVID-19 receiving ADE from other coronaviruses? Microbes Infect 2020;22(2):72–3.
41. Wang SF, Tseng SP, Yen CH, et al. Antibody-dependent SARS coronavirus infection is mediated by antibodies against spike proteins. Biochem Biophys Res Commun 2014;451(2):208–14.
42. Akbar AN, Gilroy DW. Aging immunity may exacerbate COVID-19. Science 2020; 369(6501):256–7.
43. Franceschi C, Garagnani P, Vitale G, et al. Inflammaging and "Garb-aging. Trends Endocrinol Metab TEM 2017;28(3):199–212.
44. Brodin P. Immune determinants of COVID-19 disease presentation and severity. Nat Med 2021;27(1):28–33.
45. Varikasuvu SR, Dutt N, Thangappazham B, et al. Diabetes and COVID-19: a pooled analysis related to disease severity and mortality. Prim Care Diabetes 2021;15(1):24–7.
46. Guan WJ, Liang WH, Zhao Y, et al. Comorbidity and its impact on 1590 patients with COVID-19 in China: a nationwide analysis. Eur Respir J 2020;55(5):2000547.
47. Sanyaolu A, Okorie C, Marinkovic A, et al. Comorbidity and its impact on patients with COVID-19. SN Compr Clin Med 2020;2(8):1069–76.
48. Wang B, Li R, Lu Z, et al. Does comorbidity increase the risk of patients with COVID-19: evidence from meta-analysis. Aging 2020;12(7):6049–57.
49. Imam Z, Odish F, Gill I, et al. Older age and comorbidity are independent mortality predictors in a large cohort of 1305 COVID-19 patients in Michigan, United States. J Intern Med 2020;288(4):469–76.
50. Nogueira PJ, de Araújo Nobre M, Costa A, et al. The role of health preconditions on COVID-19 deaths in Portugal: evidence from surveillance data of the first 20293 infection cases. J Clin Med 2020;9(8):2368.
51. Ye C, Zhang S, Zhang X, et al. Impact of comorbidities on patients with COVID-19: a large retrospective study in Zhejiang, China. J Med Virol 2020;92(11):2821–9.
52. Djaharuddin I, Munawwarah S, Nurulita A, et al. Comorbidities and mortality in COVID-19 patients. Gac Sanit 2021;35(Suppl 2):S530–2.
53. Sharif N, Opu RR, Ahmed SN, et al. Prevalence and impact of comorbidities on disease prognosis among patients with COVID-19 in Bangladesh: a nationwide study amid the second wave. Diabetes Metab Syndr 2021;15(4):102148.
54. Harrison SL, Fazio-Eynullayeva E, Lane DA, et al. Comorbidities associated with mortality in 31,461 adults with COVID-19 in the United States: a federated electronic medical record analysis. PLoS Med 2020;17(9):e1003321.
55. McMichael TM, Currie DW, Clark S, et al. Epidemiology of Covid-19 in a long-term care facility in King County, Washington. N Engl J Med 2020;382(21):2005–11.
56. Caballero AE, Ceriello A, Misra A, et al. COVID-19 in people living with diabetes: an international consensus. J Diabetes Complications 2020;34(9):107671.

57. Apicella M, Campopiano MC, Mantuano M, et al. COVID-19 in people with diabetes: understanding the reasons for worse outcomes. Lancet Diabetes Endocrinol 2020;8(9):782–92.

58. Fadini GP, Morieri ML, Longato E, et al. Prevalence and impact of diabetes among people infected with SARS-CoV-2. J Endocrinol Invest 2020;43(6):867–9.

59. Mithal A, Jevalikar G, Sharma R, et al. High prevalence of diabetes and other comorbidities in hospitalized patients with COVID-19 in Delhi, India, and their association with outcomes. Diabetes Metab Syndr 2021;15(1):169–75.

60. Wang Z, Du Z, Zhu F. Glycosylated hemoglobin is associated with systemic inflammation, hypercoagulability, and prognosis of COVID-19 patients. Diabetes Res Clin Pract 2020;164:108214.

61. Yan Y, Yang Y, Wang F, et al. Clinical characteristics and outcomes of patients with severe covid-19 with diabetes. BMJ Open Diabetes Res Care 2020;8(1): e001343.

62. Targher G, Mantovani A, Wang XB, et al. Patients with diabetes are at higher risk for severe illness from COVID-19. Diabetes Metab 2020;46(4):335–7.

63. Schlesinger S, Neuenschwander M, Lang A, et al. Risk phenotypes of diabetes and association with COVID-19 severity and death: a living systematic review and meta-analysis. Diabetologia 2021;64(7):1480–91.

64. Damayanthi HDWT, Prabani KIP. Nutritional determinants and COVID-19 outcomes of older patients with COVID-19: a systematic review. Arch Gerontol Geriatr 2021;95:104411.

65. Landi F, Picca A, Calvani R, et al. Anorexia of aging: assessment and management. Clin Geriatr Med 2017;33(3):315–23.

66. Recinella G, Marasco G, Serafini G, et al. Prognostic role of nutritional status in elderly patients hospitalized for COVID-19: a monocentric study. Aging Clin Exp Res 2020;32(12):2695–701.

67. Bedock D, Bel Lassen P, Mathian A, et al. Prevalence and severity of malnutrition in hospitalized COVID-19 patients. Clin Nutr ESPEN 2020;40:214–9.

68. Zuo P, Tong S, Yan Q, et al. Decreased prealbumin level is associated with increased risk for mortality in elderly hospitalized patients with COVID-19. Nutr Burbank Los Angel Cty Calif 2020;78:110930.

69. Okazaki T, Suzukamo Y, Miyatake M, et al. Respiratory muscle weakness as a risk factor for pneumonia in older people. Gerontology 2021;67(5):581–90.

70. Lidoriki I, Frountzas M, Schizas D. Could nutritional and functional status serve as prognostic factors for COVID-19 in the elderly? Med Hypotheses 2020;144: 109946.

71. Svartengren M, Falk R, Philipson K. Long-term clearance from small airways decreases with age. Eur Respir J 2005 Oct;26(4):609–15.

72. Ho JC, Chan KN, Hu WH, et al. The effect of aging on nasal mucociliary clearance, beat frequency, and ultrastructure of respiratory cilia. Am J Respir Crit Care Med 2001;163(4):983–8.

73. Martin SE, Mathur R, Marshall I, et al. The effect of age, sex, obesity and posture on upper airway size. Eur Respir J 1997;10(9):2087–90.

74. Bourgonje AR, Abdulle AE, Timens W, et al. Angiotensin-converting enzyme 2 (ACE2), SARS-CoV-2 and the pathophysiology of coronavirus disease 2019 (COVID-19). J Pathol 2020;251(3):228–48.

75. Verdecchia P, Cavallini C, Spanevello A, et al. The pivotal link between ACE2 deficiency and SARS-CoV-2 infection. Eur J Intern Med 2020;76:14–20.

76. RodriguesPrestes TR, Rocha NP, Miranda AS, et al. The anti-inflammatory potential of ACE2/angiotensin-(1-7)/Mas receptor Axis: evidence from basic and clinical research. Curr Drug Targets 2017;18(11):1301–13.
77. Gaddam RR, Chambers S, Bhatia M. ACE and ACE2 in inflammation: a tale of two enzymes. Inflamm Allergy Drug Targets 2014;13(4):224–34.
78. Schouten LRA, Helmerhorst HJF, Wagenaar GTM, et al. Age-dependent changes in the pulmonary renin-angiotensin system are associated with severity of lung injury in a model of acute lung injury in rats. Crit Care Med 2016;44(12):e1226–35.
79. AlGhatrif M, Cingolani O, Lakatta EG. The dilemma of Coronavirus Disease 2019, aging, and cardiovascular disease: insights from cardiovascular aging science. JAMA Cardiol 2020;5(7):747–8.
80. Chen J, Jiang Q, Xia X, et al. Individual variation of the SARS-CoV-2 receptor ACE2 gene expression and regulation. Aging Cell 2020;19(7):e13168.
81. Papadopoulos V, Li L, Samplaski M. Why does COVID-19 kill more elderly men than women? Is there a role for testosterone? Andrology 2021;9(1):65–72.
82. Nieschlag E. Late-onset hypogonadism: a concept comes of age. Andrology 2020;8(6):1506–11.
83. Carcaillon L, Blanco C, Alonso-Bouzón C, et al. Sex differences in the association between serum levels of testosterone and frailty in an elderly population: the Toledo Study for Healthy Aging. PloS One 2012;7(3):e32401.
84. Saad F, Gooren LJ. The role of testosterone in the etiology and treatment of obesity, the metabolic syndrome, and diabetes mellitus type 2. J Obes 2011; 2011:471584.
85. Zumoff B, Strain G, Miller L, et al. Twenty-four-hour mean plasma testosterone concentration declines with age in normal premenopausal women. J Clin Endocrinol Metab 1995;80:1429–30.
86. Davison SL, Bell R, Donath S, et al. Androgen levels in adult females: changes with age, menopause, and oophorectomy. J Clin Endocrinol Metab 2005;90(7): 3847–53.
87. Morley JE, Perry HM. Androgens and women at the menopause and beyond. J Gerontol A Biol Sci Med Sci 2003;58(5):M409–16.

Inflammaging at the Time of COVID-19

Maria Beatrice Zazzara, MD[a,1], Andrea Bellieni, MD[a,1], Riccardo Calvani, PhD[a,*],
Hélio Jose Coelho-Junior, PhD[a,b], Anna Picca, PhD[a], Emanuele Marzetti, MD, PhD[a,b]

KEYWORDS

- Inflammation • Immunosenescence • Cytokines • Older adults • SARS-CoV-2
- Long COVID • Physical activity • Diet

KEY POINTS

- Inflammaging, a state of chronic, low-grade inflammation that accompanies aging, plays a major role in the pathogenesis of most geriatric syndromes.
- Severe acute respiratory syndrome coronavirus-2 (SARS-CoV-2) infection unleashes an abnormal inflammatory response that contributes to severe coronavirus disease 2019 (COVID-19) and, possibly, long-term sequelae.
- Inflammaging and SARS-CoV-2 infection interact in an interplay that involves acute and chronic inflammation, which predisposes older adults to severe (COVID-19).
- Medications targeting inflammation pathways have proved to be effective in reducing morbidity and mortality associated with acute COVID-19.
- Lifestyle interventions (eg, physical activity and diet) can reduce chronic inflammation and may therefore counteract long-term symptom persistence.

INTRODUCTION

With more than 400 million confirmed cases and over 6 million deaths,[1] the coronavirus disease 2019 (COVID-19) pandemic, caused by the severe acute respiratory syndrome coronavirus 2 (SARS-CoV-2), has significantly affected everyone's life. Most people infected with SARS-CoV-2 have a self-limiting infection and do recover; others experience more severe disease, with 10% of patients requiring intensive care unit (ICU) admission.[2] The case-fatality rate of COVID-19 is approximately 1.5% (https://covid19.who.int/). Most COVID-19–related deaths have occurred in those 60 years and older, and an even higher mortality was registered among the oldest old (ie,

[a] Fondazione Policlinico Universitario A. Gemelli IRCCS, L.go F. Vito 1, Rome 00168, Italy;
[b] Department of Geriatrics and Orthopedics, Università Cattolica del Sacro Cuore, L.go F. Vito 1, Rome 00168, Italy
[1] Equal contribution
* Corresponding author. Center for Geriatric Medicine (Ce.M.I.), Fondazione Policlinico Universitario A. Gemelli IRCCS, L.go F. Vito 1, Rome 00168, Italy.
E-mail address: riccardo.calvani@policlinicogemelli.it

Clin Geriatr Med 38 (2022) 473–481
https://doi.org/10.1016/j.cger.2022.03.003
0749-0690/22/© 2022 Elsevier Inc. All rights reserved.

$\geq$80 years).[3] The presence of a least 1 underlying chronic condition (eg, cancer, diabetes, hypertension, obesity, cardiovascular disease, cerebrovascular disease) is a major risk factor for death.[4–6] Older adults are more susceptible to SARS-CoV-2 infection, more prone to develop severe COVID-19, and more frequently admitted to ICUs, with consequent increased mortality.[3,5]

An extraordinary proliferation of studies suggests that SARS-CoV-2 infection unleashes an abnormal inflammatory response, the so-called cytokine storm. Indeed, severe COVID-19 in hospitalized patients is characterized by high circulating levels of C-reactive protein (CRP), interleukin (IL)-6, tumor necrosis factor alpha (TNF-α), and lymphopenia.[7] The abnormal inflammatory response, along with hypercoagulability and defective viral clearance, contributes to the development of severe pneumonia and acute respiratory distress syndrome (ARDS), with subsequent end-organ damage, multiorgan system failure, and eventually death.[8] Although severe COVID-19 disproportionally affects older people, systemic inflammation during SARS-CoV-2 infection is detected in patients of all ages, including children, in whom a severe multisystem inflammatory syndrome with features of Kawasaki has been described.[9] This implies that COVID-19–induced inflammation is not per se sufficient at inducing negative health outcomes. This article provides a pathophysiologic view of COVID-19 in older adults within the frame of inflammaging, with a focus on antiinflammatory treatments for acute and postacute disease.

DISCUSSION
The Aging Process and Inflammaging

Aging is a complex phenomenon characterized by numerous changes that result from environmental, stochastic, genetic, and epigenetic events in different cell types and tissues.[10] One of the most accredited hypotheses on the pathogenesis of aging stems from the observation that older organisms tend to develop a proinflammatory status reflected by increased circulating levels of inflammatory biomolecules.[10,11] Inflammation is instrumental to combat infections or other exogen pathogens; however, when it becomes sustained and prolonged, it can be detrimental to health. The state of chronic, sterile, inflammatory process that accompanies aging is termed inflammaging[11] and is associated with a decline in the efficiency of the immune system, named immunosenescence.[12] Hence, immunosenescence and inflammaging are 2 separate but highly intertwined entities that combine to progressively reduce the immune system's ability to trigger an effective antibody and cellular response to infections and vaccinations, and are associated with increased incidence of cancer and autoimmune diseases.[13] Immunosenescence and inflammaging can be accelerated by different factors, such as persistent tissue damage, environmental stressors, unhealthy lifestyles, and social and psychological stress, and could explain differences in resistance to SARS-CoV-2 infection between younger and older adults, and genders.[14] In this complicated picture, centenarians are outliers characterized by high circulating levels of antiinflammatory biomarkers that protect them against common age-related conditions and possibly from severe COVID-19.[14] Inflammaging plays a pivotal role in most geriatric conditions, such as sarcopenia, frailty, disability, and multimorbidity, and is a major risk factor for several age-associated chronic diseases (eg, cardiovascular disease, metabolic syndrome, diabetes, cancer, autoimmune disorders, dementia),[11,15,16] all of which are linked to increased COVID-19 fatality.[4]

The mechanisms underlying this chronic inflammatory response are difficult to decipher and are still under intense investigation. The accumulation of senescent cells is one of the mechanisms implicated in the pathogenesis of chronic inflammation.[17]

Several factors contribute to cellular senescence, including oxidative stress, genomic instability, metabolic derangement, and altered proteostasis.[10] Senescence is characterized by the arrest of cell proliferation and secretion of senescence-associated secretory phenotype factors, including proinflammatory cytokines and chemokines.[11] In addition, damaged cellular and organellar components are recognized by a network of sensors and trigger further secretion of inflammatory biomolecule.[18] Other sources of inflammaging are harmful products of commensal microbes, such as oral and gut microbiota.[19] During aging, the composition of gut microbiota changes, with reduced diversity and enrichment in proinflammatory bacteria.[20] This age-related gut dysbiosis may alter the morphology and barrier properties of the intestinal mucosa with increased permeability (so-called leaky gut).[20]

Age-related changes in both the innate and adaptive immune systems play an important role in the pathophysiology of inflammaging. Declines in the number, function, and activation of cells involved in the immune response, along with the depletion of hematopoietic stem cells and alteration in the coagulation system, are major phenotypes of immunosenescence.[12] Adaptive immunity declines with age, whereas innate immunity undergoes more subtle changes that could result in mild hyperactivity.[12] Defective regulation of the complement pathways and increased activation of the coagulation system can also determine local inflammatory reactions and lead to the development of degenerative diseases.[12]

Chronic inflammation involves several cytokines, molecular pathways, effector cells, and tissue responses that appear to be shared across age-related diseases. Clinically, it is characterized by moderately increased serum levels of several inflammatory biomarkers, including CRP, IL-6, IL-18, and TNF-α.[11,21] IL-6 is considered to be the most prominent cytokine that is shared across age-related disease conditions.[21] IL-6 serum levels also predict incident disability and frailty,[22] with a risk of developing mobility disability increasing linearly for concentrations higher than 2.5 pg/mL.[23] As such, IL-6 is hallmark of chronic morbidity and a commonly used biomarker of inflammaging.[21]

Inflammaging and Coronavirus Disease 2019

Bacterial or viral infections and/or vaccinations usually cause an immune response that confers an immunologic memory. The history of the individual exposure to different antigens shapes people's so-called immunobiography and influences the degree and characteristics of the inflammatory response to a new stimulus.[24] This trained immunity often results in a more active and functional immune system.[24] Immunosenenesce and inflammaging negatively affect the immune response to pathogens, including SARS-CoV-2, which explains, at least partly, the development of more severe clinical manifestations in older adults.[25,26] In the early phases of COVID-19, infected cells release damage-associated molecular patterns (DAMPs), such as ATP and nucleic acids, which are recognized by lung epithelial and endothelial cells, and alveolar macrophages. This process triggers the production of various proinflammatory cytokines and chemokines, allowing recruitment of innate and acquired immune cells to the site of infection.[27] The activation of virus-specific CD4+ and CD8+ T cells kills infected cells. However, in the case of a dysfunctional immune response, the accumulation of immune cells in the lungs leads to the overproduction of proinflammatory cytokines, especially IL-6, causing damage to local cells and tissue, with subsequent systemic implications.[28] In older adults, a more robust activation of innate proinflammatory pathways is thought to increase the risk of severe disease.[23,26,28] In older men, IL-6 is chronically upregulated, with a higher rate of inflammaging, which might help explain the greater risk of death by COVID-19 compared with women.[28,29] Pathophysiologic pathways in COVID-19 and risk factors for negative outcomes in individuals affected by SARS-CoV-2 share several underlying mechanisms that regulate inflammation, which might affect the clinical course of COVID-19, from flulike syndrome to severe respiratory failure and death.[30] Moreover, an acute COVID-19 episode may induce accumulation of subclinical damages that predisposes to a chronic proinflammatory state, even when the episode is mild and clinically resolved with no apparent immediate consequences.[30] Indeed, a substantial share of COVID-19 survivors experience symptom persistence for weeks or months after viral clearance.[31] This condition, known as postacute COVID or long COVID, is an increasingly recognized public health issue.[32] Common long-lasting signs and symptoms include cough, fever, dyspnea, fatigue, musculoskeletal (myalgia, joint pain) and gastrointestinal complaints, and anosmia/dysgeusia.[33] In the postacute phase, some patients show an accelerated decline in physical, cognitive, and functional abilities that resembles age-related long-term impairments.[31] Evidence shows that cytokine levels are still increased in patients with long COVID and the maintenance of a low-grade chronic inflammation could be one of the mechanisms that might explain symptom persistence.[30,34,35] From this perspective, long COVID bears resemblance with postintensive care syndrome (PICS). Patients with PICS present with cognitive, psychological, and physical disabilities, and some never fully recover.[36] Physical impairment in PICS often involves muscle weakness and fatigability, and symptoms of deconditioning,[36] all cardinal features of age-related frailty and sarcopenia.[15,37] In addition, it is worth mentioning that the long-term effects of COVID-19 on health, functional status, and quality of life may be further worsened by social distancing, isolation, and financial difficulties,[38] which indicates that the management of long COVID requires comprehensive approaches similar to those developed based on the paradigm of comprehensive geriatric assessment.[39]

Inflammation as a Therapeutic Target in Coronavirus Disease 2019

Since the beginning of the pandemic, studies on COVID-19 treatments have mostly focused on quenching the uncontrolled inflammatory response. The Randomised Evaluation of COVID-19 Therapy (RECOVERY) trial has been a cornerstone in the field by showing that dexamethasone significantly reduces mortality in patients with severe COVID-19 who require supplemental oxygen.[40] Dexamethasone is a synthetic glucocorticoid with broad immunosuppressive properties, which downregulates the differentiation of B and T cells and inhibits the production of proinflammatory cytokines and chemokines.[41] Other agents targeting specifically IL-1 and IL-6 have become routinely used in the management of critical ill patients with COVID-19. Tocilizumab and sarilumab are IL-6 receptor blockers that have proven to be lifesaving in patients with COVID-19 who are severely or critically ill and are now recommended by the World Health Organization (WHO), especially when administered along with corticosteroids.[42–44] More recently, the European Medicines Agency (EMA) approved the use of anakinra, a recombinant IL-1 receptor antagonist (IL-1Ra), in patients with COVID-19 at increased risk of disease progression to respiratory failure identified by early elevation of soluble urokinase plasminogen activator receptor serum levels.[45,46] However, the use of immunosuppressants in older adults is associated with several adverse effects and can expose frail individuals to increased risk of secondary bacterial and fungal infection during hospitalization.[47–49]

In patients with long COVID, lifestyle interventions can effectively counteract chronic inflammation independent of underlying chronic conditions, and may therefore be proposed as strategies to mitigate long-term symptom persistence.[50] Physical activity and specific nutritional strategies may be especially suitable for older adults for their potential of reducing inflammaging and supporting successful immune aging.[50,51] Indeed, regular physical activity has been associated with enhanced innate and adaptive immune functions, thereby attenuating mechanisms linked to immune-senescence.[51,52] Studies have shown that physical activity improves natural killer and neutrophil function, as well as T-cell proliferation.[51,53] Furthermore, aerobic physical exercise may induce cell death in apoptosis-resistance senescent T lymphocytes and increase the pool of naive T cells.[53] Notably, physical activity reduces the expression of toll-like receptors, transmembrane glycoproteins that initiate an immune response following recognition of DAMPs or other endogenous agents, with consequent reduced secretion of proinflammatory cytokines.[51] Furthermore, physical activity promotes the secretion of controlled levels of IL-6, which stimulates the production of immune-regulatory mediators such as IL-1ra, IL-8, and IL-10, thereby regulating the balance between proinflammatory and antiinflammatory factors and contributing to the immune homeostasis.[54,55] Similar to physical activity, dietary habits play an important role in shaping the immune system, and appropriate nutritional interventions have been shown to attenuate inflammation.[51,56] Proinflammatory diets characterized by insufficient consumption of fruits, vegetables, and whole grains, and excessive use of saturated fats, meat, processed foods, and refined sugars can induce a chronic increase in inflammatory cytokine levels even in younger adults.[57] In contrast, healthy eating patterns, such as the Mediterranean diet and vegetarian diets, may ameliorate the inflammatory process and oxidative stress, maintain gut microbial eubiosis, and decrease circulating levels of inflammatory biomarkers.[56,58,59] The New Dietary Strategies Addressing the Specific Needs of the Elderly Population for Healthy Aging in Europe" (NU-AGE) project has demonstrated the feasibility of a tailored Mediterranean-like dietary pattern, specifically designed to meet dietary needs of older adults aged 65 years old and older as a comprehensive dietary strategy to reduce inflammaging and improve health and quality of life in older adults.[60] Whether such an approach may help reduce the burden of symptom persistence in older COVID-19 survivors warrants exploration.

SUMMARY

Inflammaging and SARS-CoV-2 infection interact in an interplay that involves both acute inflammation and low-grade chronic inflammation, predisposing older adults to severe COVID-19. During the acute phase, the precipitating factor is represented by an aberrant immune response characterized by the overproduction of proinflammatory cytokines. Increased cytokine levels may persist long after viral clearance and are potentially responsible for the installment of low-grade chronic inflammation and long-lasting persistence of COVID-19 symptoms. Therapeutic approaches targeting inflammation have proven to be effective in reducing mortality during an acute COVID-19 episode. However, at the time of writing, no standard treatment is available for the postacute phase. Although further research is needed, lifestyle interventions (physical activity and specific nutritional strategies) can effectively counteract chronic inflammation and may therefore be proposed as strategies to mitigate long-term symptom persistence.

CLINICS CARE POINTS

- Inflammaging along with the abnormal inflammatory response to SARS-CoV-2 predisposes older adults to severe COVID-19.

- Targeting inflammation is key during the acute phase and reduces COVID-19 lethality.
- Behavioral interventions such as physical activity and optimal diet should be recommended to counteract symptom persistence following acute COVID-19.

DISCLOSURE

The authors have nothing to disclose.

REFERENCES

1. World Health Organization. WHO coronavirus (COVID-19) dashboard. Available at: https://covid19.who.int/. Accessed February 15 2022.
2. Sun P, Qie S, Liu Z, et al. Clinical characteristics of hospitalized patients with SARS-CoV-2 infection: a single arm meta-analysis. J Med Virol 2020;92:612–7.
3. Onder G, Rezza G, Brusaferro S. Case-fatality rate and characteristics of patients dying in relation to COVID-19 in Italy. JAMA 2020;323:1775–6.
4. Guan W, Ni Z, Hu Y, et al. Clinical characteristics of coronavirus disease 2019 in China. N Engl J Med 2020;382:1708–20.
5. Du RH, Liang LR, Yang CQ, et al. Predictors of mortality for patients with COVID-19 pneumonia caused by SARS-CoV-2: a prospective cohort study. Eur Respir J 2020;55:2000524.
6. Wang L, He W, Yu X, et al. Coronavirus disease 2019 in elderly patients: characteristics and prognostic factors based on 4-week follow-up. J Infect 2020;80:639–45.
7. Fajgenbaum DC, June CH. Cytokine storm. N Engl J Med 2020;383:2255–73.
8. Jose RJ, Manuel A. COVID-19 cytokine storm: the interplay between inflammation and coagulation. Lancet Respir Med 2020;8:e46–7.
9. Verdoni L, Mazza A, Gervasoni A, et al. An outbreak of severe Kawasaki-like disease at the Italian epicentre of the SARS-CoV-2 epidemic: an observational cohort study. Lancet 2020;395:1771–8.
10. López-Otín C, Blasco MA, Partridge L, et al. The hallmarks of aging. Cell 2013;153:1194–217.
11. Franceschi C, Bonafè M, Valensin S, et al. Inflamm-aging: an evolutionary perspective on immunosenescence. Ann N Y Acad Sci 2000;908:244–54.
12. Pawelec G. Age and immunity: what is "immunosenescence". Exp Gerontol 2018;105:4–9.
13. Oh SJ, Lee JK, Shin OS. Aging and the immune system: the impact of immunosenescence on viral infection, immunity and vaccine immunogenicity. Immune Netw 2019;19:e37.
14. Domingues R, Lippi A, Setz C, et al. SARS-CoV-2, immunosenescence and inflammaging: partners in the COVID-19 crime. Aging (Albany NY) 2020;12:18778–89.
15. Ferrucci L, Fabbri E. Inflammageing: chronic inflammation in ageing, cardiovascular disease, and frailty. Nat Rev Cardiol 2018;15:505–22.
16. Franceschi C, Garagnani P, Parini P, et al. Inflammaging: a new immune-metabolic viewpoint for age-related diseases. Nat Rev Endocrinol 2018;14:576–90.
17. Campisi J, D'Adda Di Fagagna F. Cellular senescence: when bad things happen to good cells. Nat Rev Mol Cell Biol 2007;8:729–40.

18. Picca A, Calvani R, Coelho-Junior HJ, et al. Cell death and inflammation: the role of mitochondria in health and disease. Cells 2021;10:537.
19. Biagi E, Candela M, Franceschi C, et al. The aging gut microbiota: new perspectives. Ageing Res Rev 2011;10:428–9.
20. Ragonnaud E, Biragyn A. Gut microbiota as the key controllers of "healthy" aging of elderly people. Immun Ageing 2021;18:2.
21. Maggio M, Guralnik JM, Longo DL, et al. Interleukin-6 in aging and chronic disease: a magnificent pathway. J Gerontol A Biol Sci Med Sci 2006;61:575–84.
22. Soysal P, Stubbs B, Lucato P, et al. Inflammation and frailty in the elderly: a systematic review and meta-analysis. Ageing Res Rev 2016;31:1–8.
23. Ferrucci L, Harris TB, Guralnik JM, et al. Serum IL-6 level and the development of disability in older persons. J Am Geriatr Soc 1999;47:639–46.
24. Franceschi C, Salvioli S, Garagnani P, et al. Immunobiography and the heterogeneity of immune responses in the elderly: a focus on inflammaging and trained immunity. Front Immunol 2017;8:982.
25. Gensous N, Bacalini MG, Pirazzini C, et al. The epigenetic landscape of age-related diseases: the geroscience perspective. Biogerontology 2017;18:549–59.
26. Müller L, Di Benedetto S. How immunosenescence and inflammaging may contribute to hyperinflammatory syndrome in COVID-19. Int J Mol Sci 2021;22:12539.
27. Tay MZ, Poh CM, Rénia L, et al. The trinity of COVID-19: immunity, inflammation and intervention. Nat Rev Immunol 2020;20:363–74.
28. Mojtabavi H, Saghazadeh A, Rezaei N. Interleukin-6 and severe COVID-19: a systematic review and meta-analysis. Eur Cytokine Netw 2020;31:44–9.
29. Bonafè M, Olivieri F, Cavallone L, et al. A gender-dependent genetic predisposition to produce high levels of IL-6 is detrimental for longevity. Eur J Immunol 2001;31:2357–61.
30. Bektas A, Schurman SH, Franceschi C, et al. A public health perspective of aging: do hyper-inflammatory syndromes such as COVID-19, SARS, ARDS, cytokine storm syndrome, and post-ICU syndrome accelerate short- and long-term inflammaging? Immun Ageing 2020;17:23.
31. Kim Y, Bitna-Ha, Kim S-W, et al. Post-acute COVID-19 syndrome in patients after 12 months from COVID-19 infection in Korea. BMC Infect Dis 2022;22:93.
32. World Health Organization. Coronavirus disease (COVID-19): post COVID-19 condition. Available at: https://www.who.int/news-room/questions-and-answers/item/coronavirus-disease-(covid-19)-post-covid-19-condition. Accessed 15 February 2022.
33. Carfì A, Bernabei R, Landi F. Persistent symptoms in patients after acute COVID-19. JAMA 2020;324:603–5.
34. Maltezou HC, Pavli A, Tsakris A. Post-COVID syndrome: an insight on its pathogenesis. Vaccines 2021;9:497.
35. Crook H, Raza S, Nowell J, et al. Long covid - mechanisms, risk factors, and management. BMJ 2021;374:n1648.
36. Rawal G, Yadav S, Kumar R. Post-intensive care syndrome: an overview. J Transl Intern Med 2017;5:90.
37. Wilson D, Jackson T, Sapey E, et al. Frailty and sarcopenia: the potential role of an aged immune system. Ageing Res Rev 2017;36:1–10.
38. Galea S, Merchant RM, Lurie N. The mental health consequences of COVID-19 and physical distancing: the need for prevention and early intervention. JAMA Intern Med 2020;180:817–8.

39. Gemelli Against COVID-19 Post-Acute Care Study Group. Post-COVID-19 global health strategies: the need for an interdisciplinary approach. Aging Clin Exp Res 2020;32:1613–20.

40. RECOVERY Collaborative Group. Dexamethasone in hospitalized patients with Covid-19. N Engl J Med 2021;384:693–704.

41. Cain DW, Cidlowski JA. After 62 years of regulating immunity, dexamethasone meets COVID-19. Nat Rev Immunol 2020;20:587–8.

42. Lamontagne F, Agoritsas T, MacDonald H, et al. A living WHO guideline on drugs for covid-19. BMJ 2020;370:m3379.

43. Gupta S, Wang W, Hayek SS, et al. Association between early treatment with tocilizumab and mortality among critically ill patients with COVID-19. JAMA Intern Med 2021;181:41–51.

44. World Health Organization. Therapeutics and COVID-19: living guidelines. Available at. https://www.who.int/publications/i/item/WHO-2019-nCoV-therapeutics-2022.1. Accessed 15 February 2022.

45. Kyriazopoulou E, Poulakou G, Milionis H, et al. Early treatment of COVID-19 with anakinra guided by soluble urokinase plasminogen receptor plasma levels: a double-blind, randomized controlled phase 3 trial. Nat Med 2021;27:1752–60.

46. Huet T, Beaussier H, Voisin O, et al. Anakinra for severe forms of COVID-19: a cohort study. Lancet Rheumatol 2020;2:e393–400.

47. Falcone M, Tiseo G, Giordano C, et al. Predictors of hospital-acquired bacterial and fungal superinfections in COVID-19: a prospective observational study. J Antimicrob Chemother 2020;76:1078–84.

48. Peng J, Fu M, Mei H, et al. Efficacy and secondary infection risk of tocilizumab, sarilumab and anakinra in COVID-19 patients: a systematic review and meta-analysis. Rev Med Virol 2021. https://doi.org/10.1002/rmv.2295.

49. RECOVERY Collaborative Group. Tocilizumab in patients admitted to hospital with COVID-19 (RECOVERY): a randomised, controlled, open-label, platform trial. Lancet 2021;397:1637–45.

50. Woods JA, Hutchinson NT, Powers SK, et al. The COVID-19 pandemic and physical activity. Sport Med Heal Sci 2020;2:55–64.

51. Weyh C, Krüger K, Strasser B. Physical activity and diet shape the immune system during aging. Nutrients 2020;12:622.

52. Simpson RJ, Lowder TW, Spielmann G, et al. Exercise and the aging immune system. Ageing Res Rev 2012;11:404–20.

53. Tylutka A, Morawin B, Gramacki A, et al. Lifestyle exercise attenuates immunosenescence; flow cytometry analysis. BMC Geriatr 2021;21:200.

54. Scheller J, Chalaris A, Schmidt-Arras D, et al. The pro- and anti-inflammatory properties of the cytokine interleukin-6. Biochim Biophys Acta 2011;1813:878.

55. Starkie R, Ostrowski SR, Jauffred S, et al. Exercise and IL-6 infusion inhibit endotoxin-induced TNF-alpha production in humans. FASEB J 2003;17:884–6.

56. Santoro A, Pini E, Scurti M, et al. Combating inflammaging through a Mediterranean whole diet approach: the NU-AGE project's conceptual framework and design. Mech Ageing Dev 2014;136–7.

57. Cervo MMC, Scott D, Seibel MJ, et al. Proinflammatory diet increases circulating inflammatory biomarkers and falls risk in community-dwelling older men. J Nutr 2020;150:373–81.

58. Wawrzyniak-Gramacka E, Hertmanowska N, Tylutka A, et al. The association of anti-inflammatory diet ingredients and lifestyle exercise with inflammaging. Nutrients 2021;13:3696.

59. Haghighatdoost F, Bellissimo N, Totosy De Zepetnek JO, et al. Association of vegetarian diet with inflammatory biomarkers: a systematic review and meta-analysis of observational studies. Public Health Nutr 2017;20:2713–21.
60. Berendsen AAM, van de Rest O, Feskens EJM, et al. Changes in dietary intake and adherence to the NU-AGE diet following a one-year dietary intervention among European older adults—results of the NU-AGE randomized trial. Nutrients 2018;10:1905.

Clinical Features of SARS-CoV-2 Infection in Older Adults

Francesca Remelli, MD[a],*, Stefano Volpato, MD, MPH[b], Caterina Trevisan, MD, PhD[b]

KEYWORDS

- SARS-CoV-2 • Aged • Symptoms • Symptom clusters • Comorbidity • Frailty
- Mortality

KEY POINTS

- In older people, COVID-19 clinical presentation is extremely heterogeneous, especially the atypical symptoms, as delirium, which are more likely than in younger age classes.
- COVID-19 presenting symptoms are not simply influenced by chronologic age, but by common health-related conditions in advanced age, as comorbidity and frailty.
- COVID-19 symptoms tend to aggregate in clusters, and this approach appears to better describe the clinical complexity of COVID-19 disease.
- The prognostic value of clinical presentation is poorly investigated: in older people, COVID-19 atypical symptoms, such as delirium and falls, seem to correlate with adverse outcomes.

INTRODUCTION

In April 2020, the SARS-CoV-2 (COVID-19) infection was declared a pandemic emergency by the World Health Organization,[1] and after 2 years, in January 2022, the virus had already caused more than 357 million confirmed cases and 5.6 million deaths globally.[2] Older people have been described as extremely vulnerable to SARS-CoV-2, reporting a high probability of adverse outcomes, such as hospitalization, intensive care unit admission, and mortality.[3] In the first phases of the pandemic, in older patients the fatality rate was almost 8 times higher than in younger age groups.[4] Although advanced age has been correlated with higher mortality risk, the presence of specific health-related and clinical conditions (ie, multimorbidity, disability, and frailty), common in older people, may explain the main age-related differences in susceptibility

Funded by: ITALYLETR.
a Department of Medical Science, University of Ferrara, Via Aldo Moro 8, 44124, Ferrara, ITALY;
b Azienda Ospedaliero-Universitaria di Ferrara, Via Aldo Moro 8, 44124, Ferrara, ITALY
* Corresponding author.
E-mail addresses: francesca.remelli@unife.it (F.R.); vlt@unife.it (S.V.); caterina.trevisan@unife.it (C.T.)

during SARS-CoV-2 infection.[5,6] Moreover, these conditions could also modify the clinical presentation of COVID-19, with a higher frequency of atypical symptoms and signs in older than younger age, such as hyporexia and delirium.[7]

This narrative review aims to describe the current knowledge on the clinical features of SARS-CoV-2 infection in older adults, focusing on the heterogeneity of clinical presentation and the health-related conditions that might determine a different clinical picture of this disease in advanced age. Moreover, the authors discuss the prognostic value of specific symptoms at COVID-19 presentation in older people.

HETEROGENEITY OF CLINICAL PRESENTATION OF COVID-19 DISEASE

The clinical presentation of COVID-19 disease is extremely heterogeneous (**Fig. 1**): in a Cochrane systematic review published in 2020, up to 27 symptoms and signs of SARS-CoV-2 infection were described.[8] Based on the current literature, however, it is still unclear whether this high symptoms variability depends exclusively on the characteristics of the virus or, in addition to age and sex, also on the presence of the host's health-related conditions, such as comorbidities, disability, and frailty.[7] Among patients with COVID-19 infection, the most commonly reported symptoms were fever, cough, and dyspnea; other frequent symptoms were headache, sore throat, fatigue, myalgia, gastrointestinal symptoms (such as nausea, vomiting, and diarrhea), anosmia, and ageusia.[9] Of note, in studies of older patients, anosmia and ageusia have been described more rarely, probably because they are poorly reported by the patient, as a consequence of cognitive decline, age-related sensory impairments, and because of the presence of the confounding effect of medications taken.[10] In addition, the prevalence of asymptomatic and paucisymptomatic patients is not irrelevant and may hamper the application of measures to contain the virus's diffusion.[2] A retrospective study on 141 individuals aged 50 years or older with SARS-CoV-2 infection confirmed that also in older people the most common clinical presentation of COVID-19 disease included typical symptoms, especially fever (79.5%), cough (61.4%), and dyspnea (31.8%) for those between 65 and 79 years; and fever (75.0%), cough (43.8%), dyspnea (25.5%), and fatigue (25.5%) for those aged 80 years and over.[11] Indeed, in advanced age, the variability in the clinical presentation of COVID-19 is wider owing to the higher prevalence of atypical symptoms and signs, such as gastrointestinal ones (nausea,

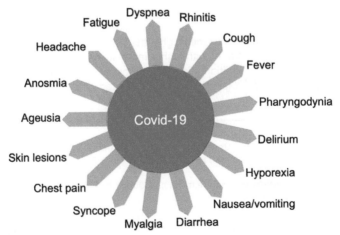

Fig. 1. Symptoms and signs of SARS-CoV-2 infection.

vomiting, and diarrhea), hyporexia, delirium, and falls.[12,13] These findings confirm previous studies that focused on the clinical presentation of common diseases in geriatric patients and observed that about one-third of older individuals admitted to the Emergency Department (ED) had atypical symptoms of the underlying disease, with the absence of fever being the most common described atypia.[14]

AGE-RELATED DIFFERENCES IN CLINICAL FEATURES

Age-related differences in the clinical presentation of COVID-19 have been widely described across the literature of the last 2 years.[15,16] In a multicenter study conducted on 107 hospitalized individuals ≥60 years old with SARS-CoV-2 infection, the oldest group of patients (>75 years old) was more likely to present atypical symptoms, such as apyrexia and hyporexia, than the youngest one. Of note, however, the most frequent clinical presentation of COVID-19 disease was characterized by typical symptoms, including fever and cough, in both age classes.[15] For example, a study sample of 788 people with COVID-19, of which more than 80% were middle-aged adults, provided similar results, and the most reported presenting symptoms on hospital admission were typical (ie, fever and dyspnea).[17] Consistently, several studies highlighted the presence of opposite trends in the frequency of typical and atypical symptoms across age classes[13,16,18]: atypical symptoms became more likely with increasing age with a parallel reduction in typical ones, although the latter remained the most frequent within the single age classes. Among atypical clinical presentations, Martín-Sánchez and colleagues[13] showed that older individuals with COVID-19 presented a higher rate of confusion (5.7% vs 0.3%) and presyncope or syncope (7.9% vs 2.4%) than adults at ED admission. The prevalence of confusion at COVID-19 onset reaches 11.7% in a sample of 103 older patients aged ≥80 years.[18] Like other infections,[19] the risk of developing delirium was higher in patients with SARS-CoV-2 infection aged 80 years and over than those 70 to 79 years old (28.4% vs 21.4%).[20] As mentioned above, when compared with older people, middle-aged adults showed atypical signs of COVID-19 disease more rarely, except for gastrointestinal symptoms. Indeed, in a prospective study performed in China in 2020 on young adults with suspected SARS-CoV-2 pneumonia, only vomiting and abdominal pain were described as atypical clinical presentations of the disease,[21] whereas no atypical signs were reported in other works involving adult individuals.[22] Of note, because of the young age of both samples (37 and 46.7 years old, respectively), no associated comorbidities were described.[21,22]

FACTORS INFLUENCING COVID-19 CLINICAL PRESENTATION

Whether the peculiar clinical features of COVID-19 in older people exclusively depends on advanced age, or rather on the presence of health-related conditions, common in geriatric individuals, such as comorbidities, motor disability, and frailty, is still uncertain. Indeed, several studies showed that older people with COVID-19 can develop different clinical pictures and degrees of severity of the disease, also within the same age class (**Table 1**).[11,23–25] In a mentioned study conducted on older patients with COVID-19,[15] almost 20% of the enrolled populations reported several complications of COVID-19 disease during their hospital stay, including acute respiratory distress syndrome, sepsis, acute renal failure, and acute heart failure. Regardless of age, for example, important clinical differences were reported based on sex, inasmuch as men more frequently develop severe COVID-19 disease than women.[26]

Moreover, a widespread hypothesis supported by the scientific community is that the presence of typical geriatric syndromes (eg, multimorbidity, disability) can

Table 1
Studies about clinical features of COVID-19 disease

Author/Year	Cohort (Country)	Study Design (Duration)	Population Characteristics	Age (y)	Sex (F)	SARS-CoV-2 Patients	3 Most Frequent Comorbidity	3 Most Frequent Symptoms and Signs of Presentation of COVID-19	Atypical Symptom of Presentation	Mortality	Conclusions
Ai et al,[21] 2020	China	Prospective (3 wk)	53 individuals with suspected SARS-CoV-2 pneumonia	COVID-19 patients: median 37.0 (IQR 33.75–50.5) Non-COVID-19 patients: median 39.0 (IQR 30.5–43.0)	50.9%	37.7%	N/A	Fever (80%) Cough (55%) Diarrhea (15%) and headache (15%)	Nausea/vomiting (5%) Abdominal pain (5%)	N/A	Symptoms were not specific for the diagnosis of COVID-19, because also similar to other viral pneumonia
Andrés-Esteban et al,[37] 2021	Spain	Retrospective (2 wk)	254 individuals ≥65 y with SARS-CoV-2 infection	Robust patients: median 69.5 (IQR 55.0–79.0) Prefrail patients: median 76.0 (IQR 66.5–82.5) Frail patients: median 81.5 (IQR 72.0–87.5)	37.8%	100%	Hypertension (35.5%) Diabetes (17.5%) Cardiomyopathy (17.2%)	Cough (56.2%) Fever (53.6%) Dyspnea (34.5%)	Diarrhea (12.5%) Nausea/vomiting (11.1%) Abdominal pain (6.1%)	27.6%	Frailty was associated with adverse outcomes, as death, in older people with COVID-19
Annweiler et al,[20] 2020	France	Cross-sectional	103 individuals ≥70 y with SARS-CoV-2 infection	Mean 84.7 (SD ± 7.0)	54.7%	100%	Hypertension (66.3%) Cardiomyopathy (45.0%) Dementia (38.0%)	Fever (77.4%) Cough (58.9%) Polypnea (39.9%)	Delirium (26.7%) Diarrhea (21.8%) Falls (18.7%) Nausea/vomiting (6.2%)	N/A	Like in young adults, in older people the clinical presentation of COVID-19 included general and respiratory symptoms, but also atypical signs, for example, delirium, falls, and gastrointestinal ones

Study	Country	Study design (duration)	Sample	Age			Comorbidities	Typical symptoms	Atypical symptoms	Mortality	Key findings
Bavaro et al,[39] 2020	Italy	Retrospective (4 mo)	206 individuals ≥65 y with SARS-CoV-2 infection	Median 80.0 (IQR 72.0–86.0)	52.0%	100%	Hypertension (60.0%) Cardiomyopathy (45.0%) Diabetes (24.0%)	Dyspnea (61.0%) Fever (55.0%) Cough (40.0%)	Confusion (39.0%)	23.0%	Frail older people with COVID-19 presented frequently extrapulmonary symptoms of disease, such as confusion
Chen et al,[22] 2020	China	Retrospective (5 wk)	136 individuals with suspected SARS-CoV-2 infection	COVID-19 patients: mean 42.9 (SD ± 13.3) Non-COVID-19 patients: mean 46.7 (SD ± 25.0)	38.2%	51.5%	N/A	Cough (68.6%) Fatigue (31.4%) Sore throat (12.9%)	N/A	N/A	A diagnostic model that included chest CT, clinical and blood test features resulted predictive for COVID-19 diagnosis
Chen et al,[43] 2020	China	Retrospective (6 wk)	203 individuals ≥18 y with SARS-CoV-2 infection	Median 54.0 (IQR 20.0–91.0)	46.8%	100%	Hypertension (21.2%) Diabetes (7.9%) Cardiovascular diseases (7.9%)	Fever (89.2%) Cough (60.1%) Chest distress (35.5%)	Diarrhea (4.9%) Nausea/vomiting (3.0%) Hyporexia (3.0%) Dizziness (2.0%) Abdominal pain (2.0%)	12.8%	In the subgroup of patients ≥65 y, no COVID-19 symptoms were correlated with mortality risk
Gálvez-Barrón et al,[18] 2021	Spain	Ambispective (8 wk)	103 individuals ≥80 y with SARS-CoV-2 infection	Mean 86.8 (SD ± 4.7)	59.2%	100%	Hypertension (81.6%) Dyslipidemia (40.8%) Dementia (35.0%)	Fever (68.9%) Dyspnea (60.2%) Cough (39.8%)	Diarrhea (15.5%) Confusion (11.7%)	57.3%	The typical COVID-19 presentation was less likely in the oldest-old, while the atypical symptoms were more frequently described
Gómez-Belda et al,[46] 2020	Spain	Retrospective (6 wk)	340 individuals ≥18 y with SARS-CoV-2 infection	Mean 65.5 (SD ± 15.0)	43.4%	100%	Hypertension (47.8%) Obesity (27.5%) Diabetes (17.4%)	Cough (63.2%) Fever (60.3%) Fatigue (42.9%)	Diarrhea (23.0%) Confusion (17.4%) Hyporexia (15.3%) Nausea/vomiting (11.5%)	16.2%	In patients >70 y, oxygen saturation ≤93% was associated with mortality
Guo et al,[15] 2020	China	Retrospective (4 wk)	107 individuals ≥60 y with SARS-CoV-2 infection	Median 67.0 (IQR 64.0–74.0)	54.3%	100%	Hypertension (43.8%) Diabetes (25.7%) Cardiovascular diseases (16.2%)	Fever (66.7%) Cough (64.8%) Fatigue (33.3%)	Diarrhea (9.5%) Hyporexia (8.6%) Nausea/vomiting (5.7%)	2.8% 60-d mortality	Patients >70 y showed more likely an atypical clinical presentation and complications of COVID-19 than younger patients

(continued on next page)

Table 1
(continued)

Author/Year	Cohort (Country)	Study Design (Duration)	Population Characteristics	Age (y)	Sex (F)	SARS-CoV-2 Patients	3 Most Frequent Comorbidity	3 Most Frequent Symptoms and Signs of Presentation of COVID-19	Atypical Symptom of Presentation	Mortality	Conclusions
Herwitt et al,[33] 2020	United Kingdom, Italy	Observational study (2 mo)	1.564 individuals ≥18 y with SARS-CoV-2 infection	Median 74.0 (IQR 61.0–83.0)	42.3%	100%	Hypertension (51.4%) Diabetes (26.5%) CHD (22.1%)	N/A	N/A	27.2% 60-d mortality	In hospitalized COVID-19 patients, frailty better predicted the mortality risk than age or comorbidities
Karlsson et al,[45] 2020	Denmark	Retrospective (3 mo)	102 individuals ≥80 y with SARS-CoV-2 infection	Median 84.0 (IQR 82–88)	53.0%	100%	Hypertension (53.0%) Cardiomyopathy (53.0%) Respiratory disease (45.0%)	Fever (74.0%) Cough (62.0%) Dyspnea (54.0%)	Confusion (29.0%) Difficulty walking (13.0%) Falls (8.0%)	31.4% in-hospital mortality 41.2% 30-d mortality	Older patients with atypical symptoms of COVID-19 (confusion and falls) reported higher mortality
Lian et al,[17] 2020	China	Retrospective (4 wk)	788 individuals with SARS-CoV-2 infection	Patients <60 y: mean 41.2 (SD ± 11.4) Patients ≥60 y: mean 68.3 (SD ± 7.3)	48.4%	100%	Patients <60 y: Hypertension (11.2%) Diabetes (5.0%) CLD (3.8%) Patients ≥60 y: Hypertension (55.2%) Diabetes (39.0%) CHD (4.1%)	Patients <60 y: Fever (79.9%) Cough (64.6%) Sputum production (33.1%) Patients ≥60 y: Fever (84.6%) Cough (62.5%) Dyspnea (36.0%)	Patients <60 y: Gastrointestinal symptoms (11.8%) Patients ≥60 y: Gastrointestinal symptoms (8.1%)	0% 30-d mortality	Older COVID-19 patients presented more likely fever and critical disease
Malara et al,[25] 2021	Italy	Prospective (10 mo)	586 individuals ≥60 y with suspected SARS-CoV-2 infection	COVID-19 patients: mean 85.5 (SD ± 8.1) Non-COVID-19 patients: mean 84.4 (SD ± 8.6)	COVID-19 patients: 72.7% Non-COVID-19 patients: 73.0%	35.7%	COVID-19 patients: Nervous system disorders (68.2%) Osteoarthrosis (54.1%) Hypertension (46.6%)	COVID-19 patients: Fever (74.9%) Delirium (41.2%) Sudden worsening of health status (35.0%)	Delirium (41.2%) Hyporexia (27.0%) Diarrhea (21.6%) Nausea/vomiting (7.2%) Fall (0.9%)	COVID-19 patients: 21.6% Asymptomatic non-COVID-19 patients: 1.8% Symptomatic non-COVID-19 patients: 10.8%	Comorbidities influenced the mortality in SARS-CoV-2-positive residents in long-term care, especially the presence of dementia

Marengoni et al,[35] 2020	Italy	Retrospective (5 wk)	165 individuals ≥65 y with SARS-CoV-2 infection	Mean 69.3 (SD ± 14.5)	39.4%	100%	Hypertension (59.4%) Diabetes (30.9%) Obesity (16.4%)	Fever (89.1%) Cough (50.3%) Dyspnea (42.4%)	Gastrointestinal signs (18.8%)	25.5%	Older patients already frail pre-COVID-19 reported a higher risk to die during the acute disease
Martín-Sánchez et al,[13] 2020	Spain	Retrospective (4 wk)	1379 individuals ≥18 y with SARS-CoV-2 infection	Median 63.0 (IQR 48.0–77.0)	46.4%	100%	Hypertension (40.5%) Dyslipidemia (37.9%) Diabetes (19.2%)	Fever (80.0%) Cough (71.1%) Dyspnea (33.3%)	Diarrhea (19.9%) Nausea/vomiting (9.9%) Pre/syncope (4.9%) Confusion (2.8%)	17.7% 30-d mortality	With increasing age, the frequency of atypical symptoms raised as the risk of the short-term mortality
Miles et al,[34] 2020	United Kingdom	Retrospective (4 wk)	377 individuals ≥70 y with or without SARS-CoV-2 infection	COVID-19 patients: mean 80.0 (SD ± 6.8)	38.0%	57.6%	N/A	N/A	N/A	37.7%	In hospitalized COVID-19 older patients, frailty was not a reliable prognostic factor
Niu et al,[11] 2020	China	Retrospective (5 wk)	141 individuals ≥50 y with SARS-CoV-2 infection	50–64 y: 57.5% 65–80 y: 31.2% 65–79 y: 31.2% ≥80 y: 11.3%	50.4%	100%	Patients 50–64 y: Hypertension (28.0%) COPD (12.0%) Cerebrovascular disease (12.0%) Patients ≥65 y: Hypertension (48.8%) COPD (29.0%) CHD (16.1%)	Patients 50–64 y: Fever (77.8%) Cough (45.7%) Fatigue (32.1%) Patients ≥65 y: Fever (78.3%) Cough (56.7%) Dyspnea (30%)	N/A	Patients 50–64 y: 1.2% Patients ≥65 y: 8.3%	Older patients with COVID-19 had a higher risk of severe disease and death
Rozzini et al,[19] 2020	Italy	Prospective (N/A)	14 individuals ≥70 y with SARS-CoV-2 infection developing delirium	Mean 78.2 (SD N/A)	21.4%	100%	Hypertension (85.7%) Cardiovascular diseases (64.3%) Diabetes (57.1%)	Dyspnea (85.7%) Fever (50.0%) Cough (28.6%)	Fall and syncope (7.1%)	71.0%	Delirium subtypes identified individuals with different prognosis, especially those with hypokinetic forms revealed the worst outcome

(continued on next page)

Table 1
(continued)

Author/Year	Cohort (Country)	Study Design (Duration)	Population Characteristics	Age (y)	Sex (F)	SARS-CoV-2 Patients	3 Most Frequent Comorbidity	3 Most Frequent Symptoms and Signs of Presentation of COVID-19	Atypical Symptom of Presentation	Mortality	Conclusions
Wang et al,[5] 2020	China	Retrospective (4 wk)	339 individuals ≥60 y with SARS-CoV-2 infection	Median 71.0 (IQR 65.0–76.0)	51.0%	100%	Hypertension (40.8%) Diabetes (16.0%) Cardiovascular diseases (14.2%)	Fever (92.0%) Cough (53.0%) Dyspnea (40.8%)	Diarrhea (12.7%) Nausea/vomiting (3.8%) Dizziness (3.8%)	19.2%	COVID-19 patients with comorbidities (ie, COPD, cardiovascular and cerebrovascular diseases) reported a higher risk of severe disease and death
Zazzara et al,[40] 2021	United Kingdom, Italy	Observational (4 wk)	448 individuals ≥65 y with SARS-CoV-2 infection	Hospital cohort: mean 77.9 (SD ± 6.8) Community cohort: mean 73.0 (SD ± 5.9)	36.6%	100%	Hospital cohort: Cardiovascular diseases (66.0%) Diabetes (40.4%) Respiratory disease (40.0%) Community cohort: Respiratory disease (21.0%) Diabetes (16.0%) Cardiovascular diseases (15.5%)	Hospital cohort: Cough (60.0%) Fever (39.0%) Delirium (25.2%) Community cohort: Fatigue (69.5%) Dyspnea (49.2%) Delirium (35.6%)	Hospital cohort: Delirium (25.2%) Community cohort: Delirium (35.6%)	N/A	Delirium might be the unique COVID-19 presenting symptom in older people, especially in frail patients

| Zhou et al,[44] 2020 | China | Retrospective (6 wk) | 108 individuals ≥60 y with SARS-CoV-2 infection | Survivors: mean 70.6 (SD ± 6.9) Nonsurvivors: mean 73.1 (SD ± 7.3) | 60.2% | 100% | Hypertension (59.3%) Diabetes (25.0%) CHD (21.3%) | Fever (75.9%) Cough (75.0%) Polypnea (64.8%) | Vomiting or hyporexia (35.2%) Dizziness (13.9%) Diarrhea (4.6%) Disturbance of consciousness (4.6%) | 47.2% | No differences in COVID-19 presenting symptoms were highlighted between survivors and nonsurvivors |

Abbreviations: CHD, coronary heart disease; CLD, chronic liver disease; CT, computed tomography; IQR, interquartile range; N/A, data not available; SD, standard deviation.

influence the COVID-19 clinical presentation (**Fig. 2**). Indeed, most of the hospitalized patients with COVID-19 reported more than one chronic disease (such as diabetes, hypertension, and coronary heart diseases)[27] and were more likely to develop a severe form of the disease.[24] In the study of Lian and colleagues,[17] older individuals showed a higher number of comorbidities than the younger group (55.15% vs 21.93%), as well as a greater risk to develop a critical COVID-19 disease. These findings were confirmed also by Niu and colleagues,[11] that reported a higher prevalence of severe COVID-19 disease in older patients and higher mortality among people ≥80 years old than in the 50 to 64 years olds (18.8% vs 1.2%, respectively). In a study on 319 patients with COVID-19 aged 60 years and over, comorbidities, such as chronic obstructive pulmonary disease (COPD) and cardiovascular and cerebrovascular diseases, increased the probability to develop a severe disease.[5] Finally, a similar picture was observed in 586 residents of long-term care facilities with suspected SARS-CoV-2 infection, with 88.8% of positive patients (n = 159) reporting 3 or more comorbidities, and this influenced the severity of COVID-19 disease (especially the presence of dementia).[25]

Several studies investigated the possible link between frailty and COVID-19 clinical presentation. It is widely known that in older patients the presence of frailty, either defined according to the Fried[28] or Rockwood criteria,[29] is strongly correlated with adverse outcomes.[30–32] Indeed, through the assessment of frailty, a better stratification of the individual's biological reserve and risk profile can be achieved, as compared with the simple assessment of chronologic age.[33] Therefore, several studies were conducted to evaluate the role of frailty in older patients with SARS-CoV-2 infection. Although the reported results are not uniform, most of the available studies support the usefulness to assess frailty in older people with COVID-19 disease.[33–37] In an observational study on 165 individuals with COVID-19 admitted in a Geriatrics Unit, Marengoni and colleagues[35] demonstrated that patients who were more likely to die during the hospitalization were already frail before COVID-19 onset (37.5% vs 4.1%).[35] In addition, every unit increment on the Clinical Frailty Scale (CFS)[38] was associated with a 30% increased risk of death, regardless of age. Despite some contrasting results,[34] in a multicenter study published in *Lancet* and including 1564 inpatients with COVID-19 with a mean age of 74 years, frailty was associated with an 83% increased risk of death in people with a CFS of 5 to 6, and with more

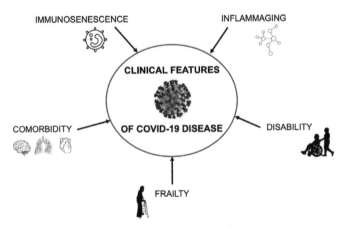

Fig. 2. Influencing factors of COVID-19 clinical presentation.

than a twofold risk in the case of a CFS of 7 to 9, regardless of age.[33] Consistent findings emerged from a prospective study on 254 older inpatients admitted for COVID-19, where frail patients were more likely to develop in-hospital delirium (43.2% vs 8.2%) and to die compared with their nonfrail counterparts.[37]

Concerning clinical presentation, Bavaro and colleagues[39] demonstrated that frail patients with COVID-19 reported a higher risk of low oxygen saturation and extrapulmonary signs at disease onset, such as electrolytes disturbances, dehydration, and confusion. In an observational study conducted on 2 cohorts in the hospital and community settings, delirium was reported as a very likely presenting symptom of COVID-19 in frail older individuals.[40] Considering that the presence of dementia is strictly connected with frailty, Annweiler and colleagues[20] showed that older patients affected by dementia had a higher risk of developing delirium at COVID-19 onset. These results were strengthened by a position paper published in 2020 by Bianchetti and colleagues,[41] where it was reported that 67% of older people with dementia developed delirium as a unique presenting symptom of COVID-19.

In conclusion, in older people, the simple chronologic age appears poorly predictive of the COVID-19 severity and health-related outcomes. For this reason, the implementation of the Comprehensive Geriatric Assessment in these patients would allow better evaluation of the presence of comorbidities, disability, and frailty, and improvement in prognostic estimation.

SYMPTOM CLUSTERS

Because of its high clinical heterogeneity, the clustering approach has been proposed to better describe the presenting symptoms of COVID-19, increase the accuracy of clinical diagnosis, and forecast the progress toward more severe forms of the disease. Indeed, some researchers observed the tendency of some symptoms and signs to aggregate, identifying specific symptom clusters of COVID-19 disease (**Table 2**).[2,10] Dixon and colleagues[2] published in March 2021 a study on community-dwelling individuals screened for SARS-CoV-2 infection, with the purpose of identifying specific symptom clusters linked to the infection presence. The investigators identified 5 symptom clusters at COVID-19 onset. Specifically, cluster 1 was characterized by the copresence of ageusia, anosmia, and fever; cluster 2 was characterized by dyspnea, cough, and chest pain; cluster 3 was characterized by asthenia, myalgia, and headache; cluster 4 was characterized by diarrhea and vomiting; and cluster 5 was characterized by rhinitis and pharyngodynia. Clusters 1 and 2 were the most strictly associated with SARS-CoV-2 infection. However, this study did not perform any subanalysis on different age groups (about one-third were >60 years old), and no information on comorbidity and preacute physical performance was reported.

In a similar study, Trevisan and colleagues[10] considered 6680 patients aged 18 years and over screened for SARS-CoV-2 infection between February and June 2020. This study aimed to identify specific symptom clusters associated with a positive SARS-CoV-2 nasopharyngeal swab and recognized 4 symptom clusters, that is, cluster 1 was characterized by flulike symptoms (rhinitis, pharyngodynia, cough, fever, myalgia, headache, gastrointestinal symptoms, anosmia/ageusia), in 40.6% of the recruited individuals; cluster 2 was characterized by generic symptoms, in 1.7% of the sample; cluster 3 was characterized by flulike + generic symptoms, in 31.5% of individuals; and cluster 4 was characterized by asymptomatic patients, involving 26.2% of the sample. At the stratified analysis, after adjusting for potential confounders (including major comorbidities), older adults belonging to the flulike

Table 2
Main characteristics of the identified studies on symptom clusters in patients with COVID-19

Author/Year	Cohort (Country)	Study Design (Duration)	Population Characteristics	Age (y)	Sex (F)	SARS-CoV-2 Patients	N. Symptom Cluster	Outcome	Results	Conclusions
Dixon et al,[2] 2021	United States	Prospective (3 mo)	8.214 individuals ≥12 y screened for SARS-CoV-2 infection	<40 y: 29.0% 40–59 y: 37.0% ≥60 y: 34.1%	55.6%	4.5%	5	SARS-CoV-2 positivity	The symptoms clusters associated with SARS-CoV-2 positivity were: (1) ageusia, anosmia, and fever; (2) dyspnea, cough, and chest pain	Anosmia and ageusia were the key symptoms for SARS-CoV-2 positivity, especially if associated with fever. The cluster characterized by severe respiratory symptoms is also strictly related to the outcome

Author	Study design	Sample	Mean age	%		Clusters	Outcome	Cluster findings	Main conclusion
Sudre et al,[42] 2021	Cross-sectional	1.653 individuals ≥16 y with SARS-CoV-2 infection	Mean (±SD) C.1: 41.1 (±11.6) C.2: 43.2 (SD ±12.1) C.3: 41.0 (SD ±12.4) C.4: 43.0 (SD ±11.9) C.5: 43.7 (SD ±13.2) C.6: 43.8 (SD ±12.2)	C.1: 70.6% C.2: 73.7% C.3: 80.1% C.4: 83.2% C.5: 72.3% C.6: 71.9%	100%	6	Need for respiratory support	C.4 (flulike symptoms), C.5 (combined respiratory symptoms), and C.6 (nonspecific symptoms) were associated with the necessity of respiratory support	Specific symptom clusters predicted the necessity of respiratory support in COVID-19 patients
Trevisan et al,[10] 2021	Cross-sectional	6.688 individuals ≥18 y screened for SARS-CoV-2 infection	Mean 47.9 (SD ±14.0)	65.7%	25.1%	4	SARS-CoV-2 positivity	Flulike symptoms cluster was associated with SARS-CoV-2 positivity	COVID-19 symptoms differently aggregated in specific clusters, influenced by age and comorbidities

Abbreviations: C.1, cluster 1; C.2, cluster 2; C.3, cluster 3; C.4, cluster 4; C.5, cluster 5; C.6, cluster 6.

symptoms cluster had a 73% higher probability of SARS-CoV-2 infection, whereas the cluster more strongly associated with a positive swab in younger people was that with flulike + generic symptoms. In both the abovementioned studies,[2,10] the investigators investigated the association between the single symptoms and the outcome identifying anosmia and ageusia as the symptoms most associated with SARS-CoV-2 infection, although the clustering approach resulted more effectively to capture the clinical complexity of COVID-19.

A third study performed using the clustering approach was conducted by Sudre and colleagues[42]: their purpose was to identify specific symptom clusters to predict the prognosis of COVID-19 disease, specifically, the necessity of respiratory support. This work is discussed in the next paragraph.

PROGNOSTIC VALUE OF COVID-19 CLINICAL PRESENTATION

Regarding the prognostic significance of COVID-19 presenting symptoms in older patients, the available literature is still not uniform. In 2 Chinese studies performed in 2020 on older individuals with SARS-CoV-2 infection, no differences in mortality were observed based on the clinical characteristics at disease onset.[43,44] On the other hand, in an Italian study conducted on 14 hospitalized older individuals with delirium during the COVID-19 disease, the investigators found that all patients who developed hypokinetic delirium died compared with the 50% of those with hyperkinetic form. These results supported the role of delirium as a negative prognostic factor in older patients with COVID-19 disease, especially the hypokinetic form.[19] These findings are consistent with those described by previous geriatric literature,[14] inasmuch delirium appeared strictly associated with a higher risk of death, regardless of clinical respiratory severity, preacute cognitive status, and motor disability. In a multicenter retrospective study in patients aged 80 years and over with COVID-19, mortality was 24% higher in those experiencing falls and 12% higher in those with confusion at the disease onset.[45] In addition to these symptoms, Gómez-Belda and colleagues[46] found that the presence of oxygen saturation $\leq$93% at COVID-19 onset was associated with increased mortality (odds ratio = 11.65, 95% confidence interval: 3.26–41.66) in patients $\geq$70 years old.

Concerning the prognostic significance of symptom clusters, to the authors' knowledge, only one study investigated the need for respiratory support (supplemental oxygen and ventilation) in patients with COVID-19.[42] This work was conducted by Sudre and colleagues[42] and included 1047 individuals with SARS-CoV-2 infection. The tendency of symptoms to aggregate in clusters was analyzed in the first 5 days from disease onset. Six symptom clusters were identified, namely: cluster 1, characterized by the presence of cough, myalgia, and anosmia; cluster 2, characterized by cough, fever, anosmia, and headache; cluster 3, characterized by gastrointestinal signs (hyporexia and diarrhea); cluster 4, characterized by flulike symptoms (cough, fever, and headache); cluster 5, characterized by combined respiratory symptoms (cough, pharyngodynia, and dyspnea); cluster 6, characterized by nonspecific symptoms (confusion and abdominal pain). When evaluating the prognostic value of symptom clusters, cluster 4 (flulike symptoms), cluster 5 (combined respiratory symptoms), and cluster 6 (nonspecific symptoms) were associated with a higher risk of needing respiratory support during the acute disease. Of note, this study involved young individuals (mean age 44 years old) and did not investigate possible age-related differences. Currently, therefore, data on the COVID-19 symptom clusters that may be more strongly associated with higher mortality are still lacking, especially as concerns older people.

FUTURE RESEARCH DIRECTIONS

Severe health-related and social effects of the SARS-CoV-2 pandemic affect especially older people, because of the high risk of social isolation, hospitalization, disability, and death. In addition, the heterogeneity of clinical presentation in this age class has often led to a delay in diagnosis, and, consequently, of treatment. Thus, based on the available studies on COVID-19 symptoms and signs in advanced age, standardized questionnaires should be created and administrated at disease onset and, in case of hospitalization, at admission; in this context, the clustering approach may help to improve the diagnostic phase of the disease. Moreover, the prognostic value of COVID-19 presenting symptoms may be extremely useful to discriminate high-risk patients; therefore, it should be deeply investigated with special attention to the older population.

SUMMARY

The COVID-19 clinical presentation is extremely heterogenous and, in older people, it is influenced not simply by chronologic age but also by common geriatric syndromes, such as multimorbidity, motor disability, and frailty. Consequently, although typical respiratory symptoms remain the most frequent clinical presentation of COVID-19 in all age classes, in older patients, atypical symptoms (including but not limited to delirium and hyporexia) are more common than in middle-aged adults and have been associated with adverse outcomes. Moreover, some studies described the tendency of COVID-19 presenting symptoms to aggregate in clusters, and this approach seems to better capture the complexity of COVID-19 disease. The prognostic value of COVID-19 symptom clusters, however, is currently poorly investigated, especially in the older population.

CLINICS CARE POINTS

- The diagnosis of COVID-19 in older patients is extremely challenging, owing to the possible presence of atypical clinical presentation, such as delirium, hyporexia, and falls.
- Older patients with comorbidity, disability, and frailty reported a higher risk of atypical presenting symptoms of COVID-19.
- The symptom cluster approach could be useful to identify COVID-19 patients with higher certainty.
- Older patients with atypical presenting symptoms and signs have a greater risk to develop a severe case of COVID-19 and to die.

DISCLOSURE

The authors have nothing to disclose.

REFERENCES

1. Word Health Organization. Coronavirus disease 2019 (COVID-19) situation report-97. Geneva: Word Health Organization; 2020.
2. Dixon BE, Wools-Kaloustian KK, Fadel WF, et al. Symptoms and symptom clusters associated with SARS-CoV-2 infection in community-based populations:

results from a statewide epidemiological study. PLoS ONE 2021;16(3 March). https://doi.org/10.1371/journal.pone.0241875.

3. Onder G, Rezza G, Brusaferro S. Case-fatality rate and characteristics of patients dying in relation to COVID-19 in Italy. JAMA - J Am Med Assoc 2020;323(18): 1775–6. https://doi.org/10.1001/jama.2020.4683.

4. Characteristics of COVID-19 patients dying in Italy. Available at: https://www. epicentro.iss.it/en/coronavirus/sars-cov-2-analysis-of-deaths.

5. Wang L, He W, Yu X, et al. Coronavirus disease 2019 in elderly patients: characteristics and prognostic factors based on 4-week follow-up. J Infect 2020;80(6): 639–45. https://doi.org/10.1016/j.jinf.2020.03.019.

6. Nickel CH, Rueegg M, Pargge H, et al. Age, comorbidity, frailty status: effects on disposition and resource allocation during the COVID-19 pandemic. Swiss Med Wkly 2020;150:20169.

7. Richardson S, Hirsch JS, Narasimhan M, et al. Presenting characteristics, comorbidities, and outcomes among 5700 patients hospitalized with COVID-19 in the New York City Area. JAMA - J Am Med Assoc 2020;323(20):2052–9. https:// doi.org/10.1001/jama.2020.6775.

8. Struyf T, Deeks JJ, Dinnes J, et al. Signs and symptoms to determine if a patient presenting in primary care or hospital outpatient settings has COVID-19 disease. Cochrane Database Syst Rev 2020;(7):2020. https://doi.org/10.1002/14651858. CD013665.

9. Yang J, Zheng Y, Gou X, et al. Prevalence of comorbidities and its effects in coronavirus disease 2019 patients: a systematic review and meta-analysis. Int J Infect Dis 2020;94:91–5. https://doi.org/10.1016/j.ijid.2020.03.017.

10. Trevisan C, Noale M, Prinelli F, et al. Age-related changes in clinical presentation of Covid-19: the EPICOVID19 web-based survey. Eur J Intern Med 2021;86:41–7. https://doi.org/10.1016/j.ejim.2021.01.028.

11. Niu S, Tian S, Lou J, et al. Clinical characteristics of older patients infected with COVID-19: a descriptive study. Arch Gerontol Geriatr 2020;89. https://doi.org/10. 1016/j.archger.2020.104058.

12. Mueller AL, Mcnamara MS, Sinclair DA. Why does COVID-19 disproportionately affect the elderly? Preprints 2020;1–32.

13. Martín-Sánchez FJ, del Toro E, Cardassay E, et al. Clinical presentation and outcome across age categories among patients with COVID-19 admitted to a Spanish Emergency Department. Eur Geriatr Med 2020;11(5):829–41. https:// doi.org/10.1007/s41999-020-00359-2.

14. Limpawattana P, Phungoen P, Mitsungnern T, et al. Atypical presentations of older adults at the emergency department and associated factors. Arch Gerontol Geriatr 2016;62:97–102.

15. Guo T, Shen Q, Guo W, et al. Clinical characteristics of elderly patients with COVID-19 in Hunan Province, China: a multicenter, retrospective study. Gerontology 2020;66(5):467–75. https://doi.org/10.1159/000508734.

16. Chow EJ, Schwartz NG, Tobolowsky FA, et al. Symptom screening at illness onset of health care personnel with SARS-CoV-2 infection in King County, Washington. JAMA - J Am Med Assoc 2020;323(20):2087–9. https://doi.org/10.1001/jama. 2020.6637.

17. Lian J, Jin X, Hao S, et al. Analysis of epidemiological and clinical features in older patients with coronavirus disease 2019 (COVID-19) outside Wuhan. Clin Infect Dis 2020;71(15):740–7. https://doi.org/10.1093/cid/ciaa242.

18. Gálvez-Barrón C, Arroyo-Huidobro M, Miñarro A, et al. COVID-19: clinical presentation and prognostic factors of severe disease and mortality in the oldest-old

population: a cohort study. Gerontology 2021;1–14. https://doi.org/10.1159/000515159.

19. Rozzini R, Bianchetti A, Mazzeo F, et al. Delirium: clinical presentation and outcomes in older COVID-19 patients. Front Psychiatry 2020;11. https://doi.org/10.3389/fpsyt.2020.586686.

20. Annweiler C, Sacco G, Salles N, et al. National French Survey of coronavirus disease (COVID-19) symptoms in people aged 70 and over. Clin Infect Dis 2021;72(3):490–4. https://doi.org/10.1093/cid/ciaa792.

21. Ai JW, Zhang HC, Xu T, et al. Optimizing diagnostic strategy for novel coronavirus pneumonia, a multi-center study in Eastern China. medRxiv 2020. https://doi.org/10.1101/2020.02.13.20022673.

22. Chen X, Tang Y, Mo Y, et al. A diagnostic model for coronavirus disease 2019 (COVID-19) based on radiological semantic and clinical features: a multi-center study. Eur Radiol 2020;30(9):4893–902. https://doi.org/10.1007/s00330-020-06829-2.

23. Yang X, Yu Y, Xu J, et al. Clinical course and outcomes of critically ill patients with SARS-CoV-2 pneumonia in Wuhan, China: a single-centered, retrospective, observational study. Lancet Respir Med 2020;8(5):475–81. https://doi.org/10.1016/S2213-2600(20)30079-5.

24. Wu Z, McGoogan JM. Characteristics of and important lessons from the coronavirus disease 2019 (COVID-19) outbreak in China: summary of a report of 72314 cases from the Chinese Center for Disease Control and Prevention. JAMA 2020;323(13):1239–42. https://doi.org/10.1001/jama.2020.2648.

25. Malara A, Noale M, Abbatecola AM, et al. Clinical features of SARS-CoV-2 infection in Italian long-term care facilities: GeroCovid LTCFs observational study. J Am Med Dir Assoc 2022;23:15–8.

26. Raparelli V, Palmieri L, Canevelli M, et al. Sex differences in clinical phenotype and transitions of care among individuals dying of COVID-19 in Italy. Biol Sex Differences 2020;11(1). https://doi.org/10.1186/s13293-020-00334-3.

27. Zhou F, Yu T, Du R, et al. Clinical course and risk factors for mortality of adult inpatients with COVID-19 in Wuhan, China: a retrospective cohort study. Lancet 2020;395(10229):1054–62. https://doi.org/10.1016/S0140-6736(20)30566-3.

28. Fried LP, Tangen CM, Walston J, et al. Frailty in older adults: evidence for a phenotype. vol. 56. 2001. Available at: https://academic.oup.com/biomedgerontology/article/56/3/M146/545770.

29. Rockwood K, Song X, MacKnight C, et al. A global clinical measure of fitness and frailty in elderly people. CMAJ 2005;173(5):489–95. https://doi.org/10.1503/cmaj.050051.

30. Guidet B, de Lange DW, Boumendil A, et al. The contribution of frailty, cognition, activity of daily life and comorbidities on outcome in acutely admitted patients over 80 years in European ICUs: the VIP2 study. Intensive Care Med 2020;46(1):57–69. https://doi.org/10.1007/s00134-019-05853-1.

31. Darvall JN, Bellomo R, Paul E, et al. Frailty in very old critically ill patients in Australia and New Zealand: a population-based cohort study. Med J Aust 2019;211(7):318–23. https://doi.org/10.5694/mja2.50329.

32. Zeng A, Song X, Dong J, et al. Mortality in relation to frailty in patients admitted to a specialized geriatric intensive care unit. Journals Gerontol - Ser A Biol Sci Med Sci 2015;70(12):1586–94. https://doi.org/10.1093/gerona/glv084.

33. Hewitt J, Carter B, Vilches-Moraga A, et al. The effect of frailty on survival in patients with COVID-19 (COPE): a multicentre, European, observational cohort

study. Lancet Public Health 2020;5(8):e444–51. https://doi.org/10.1016/S2468-2667(20)30146-8.

34. Miles A, Webb TE, Mcloughlin BC, et al. Outcomes from COVID-19 across the range of frailty: excess mortality in fitter older people. Eur Geriatr Med 2020; 11(5):851–5. https://doi.org/10.1007/s41999-020-00354-7.

35. Marengoni A, Zucchelli A, Vetrano DL, et al. Beyond chronological age: frailty and multimorbidity predict in-hospital mortality in patients with coronavirus disease 2019. Journals Gerontol - Ser A Biol Sci Med Sci 2021;76(3):E38–45. https://doi.org/10.1093/gerona/glaa291.

36. Owen RK, Conroy SP, Taub N, et al. Comparing associations between frailty and mortality in hospitalised older adults with or without COVID-19 infection: a retrospective observational study using electronic health records. Age and Ageing 2021;50(2):307–16. https://doi.org/10.1093/ageing/afaa167.

37. Andrés-Esteban EM, Quintana-Diaz M, Ramírez-Cervantes KL, et al. Outcomes of hospitalized patients with COVID-19 according to level of frailty. PeerJ 2021;9. https://doi.org/10.7717/peerj.11260.

38. Rockwood K, Theou O. Using the clinical frailty scale in allocating scarce health care resources. Can Geriatr J 2020;23(3):254–9. https://doi.org/10.5770/CGJ.23.463.

39. Bavaro DF, Diella L, Fabrizio C, et al. Peculiar clinical presentation of COVID-19 and predictors of mortality in the elderly: a multicentre retrospective cohort study. Int J Infect Dis 2021;105:709–15. https://doi.org/10.1016/j.ijid.2021.03.021.

40. Zazzara MB, Penfold RS, Roberts AL, et al. Probable delirium is a presenting symptom of COVID-19 in frail, older adults: a cohort study of 322 hospitalised and 535 community-based older adults. Age and Ageing 2021;50(1):40–8. https://doi.org/10.1093/ageing/afaa223.

41. Bianchetti A, Bellelli G, Guerini F, et al. Improving the care of older patients during the COVID-19 pandemic. Aging Clin Exp Res 2020;32(9):1883–8. https://doi.org/10.1007/s40520-020-01641-w.

42. Sudre CH, Lee KA, Ni Lochlainn M, et al. Symptom clusters COVID-19: a potential clin prediction tool COVID symptom study App. Vol 7.; 2021.

43. Chen TL, Dai Z, Mo P, et al. Clinical characteristics and outcomes of older patients with coronavirus disease 2019 (COVID-19) in Wuhan, China: a single-centered, retrospective study. Journals Gerontol - Ser A Biol Sci Med Sci 2020; 75(9):1788–95. https://doi.org/10.1093/gerona/glaa089.

44. Zhou J, Huang L, Chen J, et al. Clinical features predicting mortality risk in older patients with COVID-19. Curr Med Res Opin 2020. https://doi.org/10.1080/03007995.2020.1825365.

45. Karlsson LK, Jakobsen LH, Hollensberg L, et al. Clinical presentation and mortality in hospitalized patients aged 80+ years with COVID-19–a retrospective cohort study. Arch Gerontol Geriatr 2021;94. https://doi.org/10.1016/j.archger.2020.104335.

46. Gómez-Belda AB, Fernández-Garcés M, Mateo-Sanchis E, et al. COVID-19 in older adults: what are the differences with younger patients? Geriatr Gerontol Int 2021;21(1):60–5. https://doi.org/10.1111/ggi.14102.

Coronavirus Disease-2019 in Older People with Cognitive Impairment

Yves Rolland, MD, PhD[a,b,*], Marion Baziard, MD[a],
Adelaide De Mauleon, MD[a], Estelle Dubus, MD[a],
Pascal Saidlitz, MD[a], Maria Eugenia Soto, MD, PhD[a,b]

KEYWORDS

- COVID-19 • Dementia • Behavior disturbances • Nursing home • Ethics

KEY POINTS

- Patients suffering from dementia are at higher risk of COVID-19 infection and higher risk of severe forms and hospitalisation. There should be considered as a health priority in vaccination campaigns.Pandemia and its stay-at-home associated measures has result in higher rate behavior disturbances in demented patient that has increased burden for caregiver.
- This nursing home population accounted for about 30% of all COVID-19 related deaths in all industrialized countries and mainly among demented resident.
- Care in nursing home should be redefined according to this new situation.

Dementia affects approximately 50 million people worldwide, and this number is predicted to triple by 2050. Dementia is a disease with significant and prolonged repercussions on the patient and their family, and a huge cost for the community.[1] The combined impact of dementia and the coronavirus disease 2019 (COVID-19) pandemic have raised serious concerns about people living with dementia. Faced with the COVID-19 pandemic, the population of patients suffering from dementia has been shown to be particularly vulnerable to infection and to the severity of the disease. The application of health measures has proved particularly difficult to apply in the community as in hospital units or in nursing homes. Caregivers were challenged to ensure quality of care in difficult conditions, combining the application of

Funding sources: none.
[a] Gerontopole of Toulouse, Institute on Aging, Toulouse University Hospital (CHU Toulouse), 20 rue du Pont Saint-Pierre, Cité de la Santé, CHU de Toulouse, Toulouse 31059, France; [b] CERPOP Centre d'Epidémiologie et de Recherche en santé des POPulations UPS/INSERM UMR 1295, Toulouse, France
* Corresponding author. Gerontopole, 20 rue du Pont Saint-Pierre, Cité de la Santé, CHU de Toulouse, Toulouse 31059, France.
E-mail address: rolland.y@chu-toulouse.fr

Clin Geriatr Med 38 (2022) 501–517
https://doi.org/10.1016/j.cger.2022.03.002

appropriate health measures for the safety of all and individual respect for human dignity and ethical rules of care.

This narrative review aims to report current data on the pandemic in the population affected by dementia. After having summarized the epidemiologic data on the increased risk of infection and death in this population, this review successively discusses (i) the behavioral consequences of the social isolation and distancing measures (lockdown) such as anxiety, delirium, and depression, as well as the challenges of dealing with -wandering and pacing behaviors, (ii) current strategies, including vaccination, to face the epidemy in the dementia population, (iii) COVID-19 as a risk factor for cognitive decline and dementia, (iv) the burden of dementia for caregivers and social support during the pandemic, (v) the ethical issues, including advance directives and decision-making for hospitalization or resuscitation of dementia patient with COVID, (vi) palliative care and the critical need for advance care planning and finally (vii) care for patients with dementia living in nursing homes.

EPIDEMIOLOGY OF CORONAVIRUS DISEASE-2019 IN PATIENTS WITH DEMENTIA

From the first wave of COVID-19, the dangerousness of the COVID-19 pandemic to patients with dementia worried the medical community.[2,3] Epidemiologic data quickly highlighted the increased risk in patients suffering from dementia, not only of infection, but also of severe forms, with a frequent need for hospitalization and a high risk of death,[3–6] as well as specific complications related to their behavior disturbances.

The most recent meta-analysis on the risks associated with COVID-19 infection[3] and grouping together nearly 46,391 patients with dementia suggests that suffering from dementia increases by 2 to 3 the risk of contracting COVID-19 compared with patients of comparable age (relative risk [RR], 2.7; 95% confidence interval [CI], 1.4–5.3). Some researchers even report in studies carried out at the start of the epidemic, a significantly higher increase in risk among patients with dementia (RR, 8.5; 95% CI, 5.0–14.5).[7] This increased risk of infection can be explained by the difficulty in implementing protective measures and in particular in wearing the mask while living in an environment where many health care professionals circulate, as well as other potentially sick patients who do not observe the protective measures.[5]

A meta-analysis was published in May 2021[6] to evaluate factors associated with mortality in older adults with COVID-19. After adjustment, dementia was an independent risk factor for death (RR, 3.6; 95% CI, 2.4–5.5) that was significantly higher than other classically recognized pathologies as a risk factor for death (diabetes RR, 1.9 [95% CI, 1.5–2.3], hypertension RR, 1.3 [95% CI, 1.2–1.5], chronic obstructive pulmonary disease RR, 2.1; 95% CI, 1.5–3.1). This excess mortality of patients with dementia has been observed in particular in patients living in nursing homes.[5] Another meta-analysis published in 2021,[3] grouping 24 studies, also confirms that dementia is a risk factor for severe COVID-19 (RR, 2.6; 95% CI, 1.4–4.9), and excess mortality by COVID-19 infection (RR, 2.6; 95% CI, 2.04–3.36). In the UK, data from a large community cohort show that the risk of hospitalization for COVID-19 is approximately 3 times greater in patients with dementia than in patients without dementia.[7]

There are many reasons for the severity of the disease in patients with dementia.[8] Patients with dementia are often very old, multimorbid, and their functional reserves are low, which means that their frailty often limits their ability to cope with a potentially serious infection.[9] However, even after adjusting for these confounding factors, dementia remains a risk factor for severe COVID-19. The atypical clinical expression of patients infected with COVID-19, such as confusion, can also lead to diagnostic and therapeutic delay.[10,11] Bianchetti and colleagues[12] reported in a cohort of patients with dementia infected with COVID-19 that delirium was the most frequent presenting symptom on arrival at the hospital. Delirium is an independent, well-known risk factor for mortality and adverse outcomes in older adults. Various authors have reported that dementia was associated with more nonspecific symptoms and less clinically detected dyspnea.[12,13]

More specifically linked to Alzheimer's-type disease, carrying the ApoE4 genotype, a genetic factor associated with an increased risk of the disease, has been reported as a risk factor for more severe COVID-19 infection.[14] The modulatory function of ApoE4 on the cells of the inflammatory response, especially in the lungs, could be the explanation.[15] ApoE4 contributes to the production of proinflammatory cytokines by macrophage and may potentiate the cytokine storm seen in severe forms of COVID-19.[16]

Finally, during the pandemic, the health of patients with dementia depended more than ever on caregivers who were sometimes left out of care to limit the spread of the virus or affected by COVID-19 themselves. The impact of the reorganization of patient support as well as social isolation measures (lockdown) that are often difficult for patients to understand has potentially affected their health status[17] and help to decompensate pre-existing chronic diseases in patients with dementia more than in other populations.[18] The negative effects of the measures taken around the world to control the spread of the virus have certainly been more detrimental in patients with dementia.[9] Various studies point out that people with dementia have increased their psychiatric symptoms and behavioral manifestations caused by social isolation.[19] Loneliness at home or in nursing homes has facilitated the onset of confusion and may have resulted in agitation. Many health care providers intervene with patients with dementia living at home. The pandemic has often constrained or decreased the fragile balance of the organization of essential human care for maintaining patients at home.[17–20]

NEUROPSYCHIATRIC SYMPTOMS OF PATIENTS WITH DEMENTIA DURING THE OUTBREAK

Since the beginning of 2020, social isolation and distancing measures have been imposed on several occasions. These periods of confinement have led to a significant increase in psychological distress, such as anxiety or depression, in the general elderly population.[19] In nursing homes, residents had a higher risk of infection by COVID-19 than the population living at home and were also confronted with the absence of their relatives and limitations on activities and social interaction.[19]

Recent literature undeniably shows that the outbreak has increased neuropsychiatric symptoms in people with and without major neurocognitive impairments.[8] This increase would be more important in patients with dementia.[19] Moreover, outbreak measures have been responsible for an increase in neuropsychiatric symptoms in more than one-quarter of patients with dementia and a worsening of symptoms in more than one-half of them.[21] Whiting and colleagues[22] highlighted that the severity of neuropsychiatric symptoms measured by the Neuro-Psychiatric Inventory increased significantly since the beginning of the outbreak and especially during periods of lockdown. In patients with major neurocognitive impairment, apathy seems to be the most frequently found neuropsychiatric symptoms. Anxiety and agitation are the second most frequent neuropsychiatric symptoms.[23] In contrast, irritability, apathy, agitation, and anxiety are the most frequently worsened neuropsychiatric symptoms in this population.[21] Finally, anxiety and sleep disturbances were reported to be higher in subjects with dementia living alone at home.[24] In several studies, agitation and aggression were more severe than other neuropsychiatric symptoms, with a high impact on professional and family caregivers.[8,19,21] An Argentinean study suggests that neuropsychiatric symptoms—namely, anxiety, depression, and sleep disorders—occur more frequently in person living in the community with mild Alzheimer's disease compared with more advanced stages of the disease.[25] An Italian study focused on persons with vascular dementia living at home. It would seem that these patients have more severe neuropsychiatric symptoms overall and that the most frequently found neuropsychiatric symptoms were anxiety, delusions, hallucinations, and apathy.[26] Patients with Lewy body disease seemed to have a predilection for anxiety, sleep disorders, and, to a slightly lesser extent, hallucinations.[21] In frontotemporal lobar dementia, the most frequently increased neuropsychiatric symptoms are wandering and eating disorders.[21] In nursing homes, eating disorders have also been more frequent during the outbreak and notably during periods of lockdown.[23]

In contrast, the increase in mood disorders was found inconsistently, mainly in association with social isolation and the loss of family contacts at home or in the long-term care facilities.[27,28] Finally, psychotic disorders seemed to be the least impacted by the outbreak.[12,19,21]

The main hypotheses to explain the increase and worsening of neuropsychiatric symptoms are the social isolation and distancing measures resulting from successive lockdowns,[23] the abrupt absence of professional interventions and the outpatient care (respite day care, rehabilitation services), and, to a lesser extent, COVID-19 infection itself.[19,25,26] A small number of studies seem to suggest that delusions are the neuropsychiatric symptoms most frequently found in hospitalized patients with dementia who are infected with COVID-19.[12,19] In the long-term care facilities, social isolation, limitations of activities, in particular the sharing of meal times, and the absence of family members, explains to a large degree the increase in neuropsychiatric symptoms.[23]

Longer periods of lockdown seem to be the major cause of more severe neuropsychiatric symptoms, particularly in the apathy of individuals with Alzheimer's disease living at home.[27] Some experts have suggested that neuropsychiatric symptoms secondary to periods of lockdown may become chronic.[19]

In contrast, during these same lockdown periods, family caregivers of patients with major neurocognitive impairments also presented more neuropsychiatric symptoms, such as anxiety, mood or sleep disorders, and eating disorders.[29] One study suggests that some neuropsychiatric symptoms such as depression in informal caregivers may cause neuropsychiatric symptoms to emerge in subjects with dementia, and symptoms such as anxiety and depression in informal caregivers may exacerbate pre-existing neuropsychiatric symptoms.[30]

Finally, several studies have highlighted that the most common response to increased neuropsychiatric symptoms during lockdown and outbreak periods has been increased prescribing of psychotropic medications.[21,25-27]

IMPACT OF CORONAVIRUS DISEASE-2019 ON COGNITIVE DECLINE IN PATIENTS WITH DEMENTIA

Patients with dementia, particularly the elderly, are among the most vulnerable populations facing COVID-19 infection. This population often suffers from sensorial deficits and perception troubles, including visual and hearing difficulties, and an inability to recognize or understand their environment and thus, to adapt to changes. This factor is even more important with the mask-wearing measures. In addition, COVID-19 social isolation measures led both to a greater psychological distress and, at the same time, to a minor cognitive and functional stimulation in the patients with dementia. As a consequence, cognitive decline has been shown to be exacerbated by the pandemic.[31–33] More specifically, memory, orientation, motor abilities, and language skills seem to be the most affected cognitive domains in these patients.[34]

In contrast, it is known that COVID-19 infection may have an impact on neurological functioning, resulting in worsening cognitive decline, even in patients without dementia, and certainly in patients with dementia. The potential mechanisms underlying these symptoms are not understood fully, but are probably multifactorial, involving indirect proinflammatory general state and direct neurotrophic effect of severe acute respiratory disease coronavirus 2.[35] Neurotropism is associated with various mechanisms, including retrograde neuronal transmission via olfactory pathway, a general hematogenous spread, and the virus using immune cells as vectors.[35]

Lessons learned from this pandemic show that further crisis and emergency phases should not neglect the multiple needs of patients with neurocognitive disorders and that a special support system will be urgently necessary to be addressed to these patients to avoid a decline in cognitive functioning, a hallmark symptom of Alzheimer's disease and related disorders.

VACCINATION OF PATIENTS WITH DEMENTIA

People with dementia suffering from COVID-19 infection are a higher risk of severe forms, longer hospitalizations, and high mortality rates.[36] In contrast, social isolation and distancing, face mask, proper hand washing, and other anti–COVID-19 measures often become extremely difficult to be respected owing to patients' cognitive and behavioral disturbances.

Therefore, given these negative health outcomes and difficulties, these patients should greatly benefit from the COVID-19 vaccine, and they should be considered as a health priority in vaccination campaigns in both living settings, namely, those in the community and those in nursing homes. However, they might need the encouragement of health professionals and families to become vaccinated. Proxy and professionals' preferences regarding vaccination for this group are, therefore, extremely important to increase the use of this preventive measure.[37]

Nevertheless, concerns still arise from safety of these news vaccines in this population with neurocognitive disorders.[38]

IMPACT OF "STAY-AT-HOME MEASURES" ON PATIENTS WITH DEMENTIA

Stay-at-home measures, mainly lockdown periods and social isolation during the COVID-19 crisis, have had an important negative impact on patients with dementia. In fact, functional, cognitive, and behavioral outcomes, as well as quality of life, have worsened significantly in this vulnerable population throughout this pandemic.[8] The main reason is that patients with dementia have suffered all the collateral sides effects of COVID-19 measures; first, by canceling many ambulatory and outpatient activities and/or planned hospitalizations, these patients lacked their regular disease follow-up and care from the family doctor or at the memory specialist. In addition, decompensation of other chronic conditions or emerging acute diseases were not be able to be managed appropriately.[39] Second, all care activities provided to patients with dementia, such as daily home care, respite day care, home professionals like physiotherapist, therapist, or mobiles teams, diminished their interventions or event were disrupted because of COVID-19 measures. As consequence, patients' diseases have worsened in terms of cognitive and physical decline, as well as in behavioral and psychological disturbances. This negative impact has been also observed in caregivers, who were facing the disease alone.

However, the challenges posed by COVID-19 have led to development and innovation in terms of providing care, whether that be via telemedicine, the development of new online tools, or receiving treatment within one's home.[40] In fact, the COVID-19 pandemic has been an accelerator for the implementation of new technologies applied to the care and management of patients with dementia and their caregivers. Indeed, the implementation of teleconsultation has been a tremendous advance.[41] Patients and caregivers were extremely grateful and relieved that health professionals were still there. Although there are several limitations to teleconsultation, patients and caregivers have accepted this new way of interaction and follow-up. Currently, health professionals, mainly physicians, still use this method of care in conjunction with traditional follow-up consultations, especially in cases such as severe dementia and behavioral disorders.

For the future, this experience has opened many doors and provides new possibilities to enhance follow-up based on telehealth in conjunction with the traditional in-person consultations for patients with dementia. For example, monitoring alerts first signs of cognitive decline, or risk for falls, or risk for behavioral disturbances is an important challenge for future telemonitoring tools; the development of novel interventions or monitoring system for pharmacologic treatment can be applied to issues of tolerance and efficacy. Concerning caregivers, in the same manner, new tools addressed to them could be used to enhance their training or support. Indeed, monitoring alerts the first signs of high burden, depression, or health problems could allow preventive interventions for caregivers.

Finally, COVID-19 and these new technologies have allowed novel ways of providing care much closer to patients and caregivers, toward a home care–centered model for dementia and away from a hospital-centered model.

BURDEN OF DEMENTIA DURING CORONAVIRUS DISEASE-2019

Major neurocognitive disorders,[42] led by Alzheimer's disease,[43] are the cause, according to their definition, of a loss of independence in instrumental and fundamental activities[42] of daily living. These disorders can also be associated with behavioral disorders[44,45] as discussed elsewhere in this article. Thus, these symptoms can cause a burden on caregivers. This burden causes psychological[46–48] and physical[47] stress for caregivers, which can lead to institutionalization for patients.[49]

The COVID-19 pandemic has caused many disturbances. First, owing to the high mortality rate of COVID-19, especially in the elderly,[50] and the lack of an effective specific molecule or vaccine, most countries implemented social distancing and home confinement measures to avoid gatherings and, thus, the spread of the virus.[51] Second, the health situation has impacted indirectly formal and informal caregivers and the health system they rely on. Indeed, care procedures considered nonurgent were suspended temporarily,[52] centers were closed,[53–55] and health professionals were sick or had to modify their schedules to cope with their own difficulties; therefore, telemedicine was promoted.[40,56]

In the general population, these measures contributed to mental health problems,[57] a decrease in physical activity, and thus an increase in sedentary behavior.[58] For people with major neurocognitive disorders, it may have been difficult to understand the health situation and, more specifically, to implement social distancing measures,[59] which may have led to an increase in behavioral problems and a loss of functional independence in the activities of daily living.[33,60] The caregivers, sometimes still working, have had to adapt their workstation, for example, by teleworking. Most of the time, they have had to cope with increased financial stress while continuing to manage their family and their sick loved one. Indeed, several studies show that the health situation related to COVID-19 caused an increase in caregiver burden and a decrease in their well-being,[33] an increase in caregiver exhaustion,[32] an increase in stress levels[61,62] with an increase in anxiety,[63] particularly about transmitting the infection to their relative,[53] and finally an increase in depressive symptoms.[64] In addition, older caregivers seem to have been the most vulnerable to this increase in stress.[53] Finally, the burden was greater the more advanced the stage of neurocognitive impairment was.[65]

To decrease the burden on the caregiver, several researchers have worked on proposing concrete solutions. For example, the work of Ercoli's team has put forward 3 approaches to limit the stress and burden related to COVID-19: first, education about COVID-19. The second approach is stress prevention by maintaining daily routines, especially sleep, daily physical activity, and communication with the ill family member, as also shown by the Goodman–Casanova team. Finally, the last axis is based on the self-care of caregivers, notably through monitoring their mental health, participation in discussion groups, and mindfulness meditation.[24,66]

Other studies emphasize the use of telemedicine for patients and their caregivers. Indeed, studies have shown the effect of teleconsultation on the well-being of patients suffering from dementia and their caregivers.[56]

ETHICAL ISSUES IN PATIENTS WITH COGNITIVE IMPAIRMENT

The COVID-19 pandemic, both through health and psychological effects, and through the impact of control measures, raises many ethical questions in the care of patients with cognitive impairment. Some bibliographic sources have been interested in ethical questions and their main pillars: beneficence, nonmaleficence, justice, autonomy, and dignity.[67]

Impact on the Care of Elderly Patients with Cognitive Disorders

Cognitive impairment represents a risk factor for a serious form of infection with severe acute respiratory syndrome coronavirus 2[68] for many reasons: associated comorbidities, drug-related causes, delayed or sometimes inappropriate treatments, and behavioral disorders that make care complex. However, some less obvious factors may be involved as well, including socioeconomic conditions and increasing disparities.[69]

In this sense, the ethical discussion concerning sometimes high-acuity care (high-flow oxygen therapy, transfer to hospital or intensive care unit) must consider the presence of cognitive impairment, and sometimes associated neuropsychiatric symptoms. It is the patient's prognosis, and not their age alone, that must be taken into account in these discussions.[70] The difficulties in obtaining the consent of persons with cognitive impairment, in the discussion concerning the continuation of high-acuity care, highlights the importance of seeking upstream the designation of a medical power of attorney and the discussion and creation of advance directives.[71] Some recommendations have been made to facilitate the management of patients with cognitive impairment in the context of the COVID-19 pandemic,[72] particularly for palliative support, stressing the need for collegiality and interdisciplinary collaboration.

Psychological Impact of the Pandemic and Health Measures

Social isolation and a reduction in outside healthcare and support workers available for people living at home may have contributed to greater psychological weakness, more frequent mood disorders, or even to the increase in certain neuropsychiatric symptoms linked to neurological disease.[23] Likewise, social distancing measures, starting with wearing a mask, can make it difficult to communicate with people with cognitive impairment. Nonverbal communication and the use of appropriate face masks can be of great help in promoting understanding despite cognitive disorders.[5]

In long-term care units, residents regularly experience periods of isolation and fewer outside interventions or activities. Caregivers in these facilities observed changes in the mental health of residents with cognitive impairment. The health measures in these care settings, in particular the isolation of residents who sometimes cannot give informed consent to these measures, require them to be adapted to the well-being and safety of the patients.[73] Reflection on the appropriate isolation measures for the epidemic situation, as well as the adaptation of existing legislative texts, remains necessary in this context.[74]

Development of Alternatives and New Care Methods

With the pandemic and the health containment measures, we have seen the development of new activities and the acceleration of other measures previously less developed. This is particularly the case with telemedicine, which has made it possible to continue medical support for isolated people or with cognitive disorders, living at home or in institutions.[71,75,76]

We have also seen, for elderly people with COVID-19 requiring complex medical care (oxygen therapy) who were not hospitalized, the development of hospital levels of care at home significantly increased during this period.

PALLIATIVE CARE IN PATIENTS WITH COGNITIVE IMPAIRMENT

Patients with dementia have an increased risk of developing COVID-19 infection. Moreover, all-cause dementia is considered a comorbidity associated with an increased risk of mortality.[77,78] In this context, there has been a significant use of palliative care in the management of patients with dementia with COVID-19.

Palliative care is a comprehensive and individualized care that should begin early in the course of any life-limiting disease.[79] During the pandemic, there was a lack of hospital beds, and palliative care had to be implemented in long-term care units.[80] This situation led to ethical discussions in the institutions and caused distress among the staff and relatives.[72] Care choices, if they were not anticipated, had to be made in a less than ideal context. Overload caregivers working during this period, the shortage of health care professionals, the absence of families and their doctor (prohibited from entering the nursing homes), and the low availability of beds at the hospital and of hospital professionals forced health care professionals in nursing homes to endorse complicated ethical choices, for which they were sometimes not prepared. This situation has revealed the importance of palliative care networks and the need for nursing homes to work on advanced directives and procedures regarding end-of-life and palliative care management.

The therapeutic means used in the management of respiratory symptoms are preferably opioids and oxygen therapy in case of hypoxemia. For behavioral disorders such as agitation and anxiety, the recommended treatment is benzodiazepines.[81] These behavioral disorders can be increased by isolation or restrictions on visits.[82] This also required care and support for the families, especially because isolation measures had to be respected.[83]

This management of the COVID-19 pandemic highlighted a lack of early discussion about the life plans of nursing homes patients. Kaasalainen and colleagues[83] established recommendations for end-of-life and palliative care management for patients with dementia during the COVID-19 crisis and beyond. In this article, the Alzheimer Society of Canada proposes a coordinated multistep approach to improve palliative and end-of-life care for people with dementia in nursing homes during the COVID-19 pandemic.

CARE FOR THE PATIENT WITH DEMENTIA IN A NURSING HOME DURING THE PANDEMIC

COVID-19 infection is a disease mainly affecting elderly people and, among them, the most vulnerable living in nursing homes. Some data demonstrate the severity of the epidemic in nursing homes: Across the United States, approximately 1.4 million people live in nursing homes, or approximately 0.4% of the 330 million Americans. This nursing home population accounted for more than 180,000 COVID-19 deaths, or about 30% of all COVID-19–related deaths in the United States. In France, approximately 1% of the general population live in nursing homes. This small group has also accumulated, as in other European and industrialized countries, approximately 30% of all COVID-19 deaths.[84,85] The drama experienced by the nursing homes can be explained by the physical regrouping of people; their very old age, their great vulnerability owing to their immunosuppression, their multimorbidity, and, in particular, a prevalence in nursing homes of more than 50% of residents with dementia. Dementia has been repeatedly reported as an important risk factor for deaths related to COVID-19. This factor has led to the completion of numerous studies on the COVID-19 epidemic in nursing homes.[86–88]

The scientific literature quickly highlighted the challenge of providing care for residents with dementia, both to limit the risk of the virus spreading in the nursing homes and also to ensure quality care for this population.[89] Various authors highlight the difficulty of taking care of residents treated with psychotropic drugs during the epidemic,[72] as well as those with cognitive impairment.[67] The increased risk of COVID-19 in patients with dementia living in nursing homes and their roommate or environment, who are often also affected by dementia, is explained in particular by their great difficulty in applying barrier measures. All the unfavorable components of a severe and difficult to control epidemic are present in patients with dementia living in nursing homes.[90,91]

The use of masks, room isolation, and decreased mobility in the nursing homes quickly proved to be complicated to understand by the residents and unrealistic to apply by the nursing homes staff among the most impaired residents, especially those exhibiting wandering behavior.[92,93] Distancing (quarantine, isolation, cohorting) are effective strategies for fighting against pandemics,[94] but it has been difficult to implement effectively in nursing homes, especially for residents with dementia.[73] Moreover, the side effects of recommendations against the spread of COVID-19 in nursing homes were particularly significant among residents with dementia. Indeed, recommendations based on barrier measures (social distancing, limiting visits, especially from families) decreased the possibilities for social interactions, physical activity, and other nonpharmacological measures for decreasing psychobehavioral disorders. These measures were associated with an increase in anxiety, loneliness, and depressive symptoms in residents with cognitive impairment, for whom the explanations given were not understood.[39,93] Likewise, the strict application of social isolation and distancing measures have sometimes increased the use of physical restraints or the use of psychotropic drugs.[39,73,93]

For the family, restricting visits has generated concern about the consequences of loneliness on their loved ones.[95] The involvement of families in providing palliative care support to their loved ones suffering from dementia during the epidemic has been hampered owing to the constraints of nursing homes visits.[96] Articles on this subject highlight the difficulties encountered by nursing home staff in discussing advance directives for hospitalization or resuscitation with patients with dementia who do not understand the situation and with referring families who were prohibited from visiting their loved ones because of the pandemic.[72] Despite these constraints, the pandemic period seems to have encouraged team discussions and discussions with residents' representatives on advance directives in nursing homes.[97] Despite the frequency of this situation, a recent review of the literature shows that work on the specific challenges of supporting the end of life of residents with dementia duly infected with COVID-19 is lacking. The ethical dimensions, and the cultural and spiritual aspects of the accompaniment of residents, their relatives, and their care teams have so far been little studied.[72] Recommendations for nursing staff on providing palliative care for people with dementia in long-term care facilities have been proposed.[72]

SUMMARY

The epidemic was indicative of the limits of organizations caring for the elderly with dementia, but also of the capacity for innovation and resilience of caregivers and families.

The design of nursing homes, often accommodating large number of residents at a single site, most of them with dementia and unable to understand and apply social isolation and distancing measures, has contributed to the problem of COVID-19 infection. The difficulties caused by double occupancy rooms of large and sometime poorly ventilated institutions should lead to a reexamination of the nursing homes of tomorrow.[98] Cohorting has often been difficult to organize in nursing homes clusters owing to architectural constraints. Research should question the applicability of barrier measures, particularly in specialized Alzheimer's units and in the particular situation of wandering patients.[99,100] The challenge is considerable; all the previous data argue for an increase in social interactions in nursing homes.[101]

A major problem in the community and in nursing homes has been the isolation of patients with dementia and their disconnection from their families and other loved ones. The multiple innovations initiated by caregivers or families must be sustained, improved, and evaluated in future research.[102] The epidemic will have had the outcome of showing everyone the benefits of telemedicine, so far in its infancy in many health care structures, in the prevention of avoidable hospitalizations, and in the improvement of care.[103] Once the epidemic has passed, it will be up to us to perpetuate these practices for the good of patients with dementia.

Data from the literature show that the consequences of the pandemic in patients with dementia go far beyond the risks of COVID-19 pneumonia. It seems that the quality of care given to nursing homes residents has been particularly complex to maintain.[67,91]

The long-term consequences of the decline in physical activity in patients with dementia, most often at high risk of motor functional decline and falls, will be assessed in future work. Current data are already showing the impact on the well-being, cognitive decline, and loss of functional abilities of the most fragile patients.[104] The experience acquired on the evaluation of the benefit–risk balance of barrier measures and their ethical dimensions will be taken into consideration for future years and in the event of a new epidemic. Longitudinal studies will also be needed to assess the neurocognitive consequences associated with COVID-19 in the long term.[105]

Although no study has looked specifically at the efficacy of vaccination in patients with dementia, or in the most fragile patients,[106,107] observational data, particularly in nursing homes, have confirmed the benefits of vaccination in this population without a greater number of adverse effects than in the rest of the population. This finding is reassuring, but testifies to our difficulty in carrying out research and providing solid scientific data on the patients most affected by the epidemic.

Health care teams, such as in Singapore (no doubt more accustomed to using new technologies), report innovative initiatives[108] for patients with dementia, such as physical exercise programs, as well as dementia patient care programs offered by the ADA such as "Stay Home Fun," which contains fun activities such as karaoke, bingo, cooking, and singing.[109] These initiatives should be made known to everyone.

In conclusion, we cannot ignore the impact of the COVID-19 pandemic on the progress of therapeutic clinical research on Alzheimer's disease, which has most often been stopped for safety reasons during the pandemic. The delay and loss of opportunity for innovative drugs for participants and future patients as well as the loss of research money for the disease is also a tragedy. This situation should inspire us to have a procedure allowing the pursuit of remote research in such a situation. In this field of research, this epidemic should lead us to be innovative by using new methods and virtual remote evaluation devices that are efficient and validated.[39]

CLINICS CARE POINTS

- Significant attention must be paid to demented patients (application of health recommendations, vaccination) to limit their risk of COVID-19 infection.
- A regular exhaustion assessment of caregivers must be carried out in order to provide the appropriate aids.
- The training of nursing home care teams in epidemic situations must be reinforced in the training programs.
- The pandemic has underlined the importance of initiating ethical reflections in retirement homes.
- Given the consequences of containment measures on the behavior of demented patients, the assessment of the risk/benefit balance must be carried out regularly.

CONFLICTS OF INTEREST

The authors have nothing to disclose.

REFERENCES

1. World Alzheimer Report 2018 - The state of the art of dementia research: new frontiers. NEW Front.:48.
2. July J, Pranata R. Prevalence of dementia and its impact on mortality in patients with coronavirus disease 2019: a systematic review and meta-analysis. Geriatr Gerontol Int 2021;21(2):172–7.
3. Hariyanto TI, Putri C, Arisa J, et al. Dementia and outcomes from coronavirus disease 2019 (COVID-19) pneumonia: a systematic review and meta-analysis. Arch Gerontol Geriatr 2021;93:104299. https://doi.org/10.1016/j.archger.2020.104299.
4. Rutten JJS, van Loon AM, van Kooten J, et al. Clinical Suspicion of COVID-19 in nursing home residents: symptoms and mortality risk factors. J Am Med Dir Assoc 2020;21(12):1791–7.e1.

5. Gil R, Arroyo-Anlló EM. Alzheimer's disease and face masks in times of COVID-19. J Alzheimers Dis JAD 2021;79(1):9–14.

6. Alves VP, Casemiro FG, Araujo BG de, et al. Factors associated with mortality among elderly people in the COVID-19 pandemic (SARS-CoV-2): a systematic review and meta-analysis. Int J Environ Res Public Health 2021;18(15):8008.

7. Atkins JL, Masoli JAH, Delgado J, et al. Preexisting comorbidities predicting COVID-19 and mortality in the UK Biobank community cohort. Newman AB. J Gerontol Ser A 2020;75(11):2224–30.

8. Numbers K, Brodaty H. The effects of the COVID-19 pandemic on people with dementia. Nat Rev Neurol 2021;17(2):69–70.

9. Bonanad C, García-Blas S, Tarazona-Santabalbina F, et al. The effect of age on mortality in patients with COVID-19: a meta-analysis with 611,583 subjects. J Am Med Dir Assoc 2020;21(7):915–8.

10. Pranata R, Huang I, Lim MA, et al. Delirium and mortality in coronavirus disease 2019 (COVID-19) – a systematic review and meta-analysis. Arch Gerontol Geriatr 2021;95:104388. https://doi.org/10.1016/j.archger.2021.104388.

11. Hariyanto TI, Putri C, Hananto JE, et al. Delirium is a good predictor for poor outcomes from coronavirus disease 2019 (COVID-19) pneumonia: a systematic review, meta-analysis, and meta-regression. J Psychiatr Res 2021;142:361–8. https://doi.org/10.1016/j.jpsychires.2021.08.031.

12. Bianchetti A, Rozzini R, Guerini F, et al. Clinical presentation of COVID19 in dementia patients. J Nutr Health Aging 2020;24(6):560–2.

13. Poloni TE, Carlos AF, Cairati M, et al. Prevalence and prognostic value of Delirium as the initial presentation of COVID-19 in the elderly with dementia: an Italian retrospective study. EClinicalMedicine 2020;26:100490. https://doi.org/10.1016/j.eclinm.2020.100490.

14. Kuo CL, Pilling LC, Atkins JL, et al. ApoE e4e4 Genotype and Mortality With COVID-19 in UK Biobank. Newman AB. J Gerontol Ser A 2020;75(9):1801–3.

15. Gordon EM, Yao X, Xu H, et al. Apolipoprotein E is a concentration-dependent pulmonary danger signal that activates the NLRP3 inflammasome and IL-1β secretion by bronchoalveolar fluid macrophages from asthmatic subjects. J Allergy Clin Immunol 2019;144(2):426–41.e3.

16. Verkhratsky A, Li Q, Melino S, et al. Can COVID-19 pandemic boost the epidemic of neurodegenerative diseases? Biol Direct 2020;15(1):28.

17. Jones A, Maclagan LC, Schumacher C, et al. Impact of the COVID-19 pandemic on home care services among community-dwelling adults with dementia. J Am Med Dir Assoc 2021;22(11):2258–62.e1.

18. Dang S, Penney LS, Trivedi R, et al. Caring for caregivers during COVID-19. J Am Geriatr Soc 2020;68(10):2197–201.

19. Manca R, De Marco M, Venneri A. The impact of COVID-19 infection and Enforced prolonged social isolation on neuropsychiatric symptoms in older adults with and without dementia: a review. Front Psychiatry 2020;11:585540. https://doi.org/10.3389/fpsyt.2020.585540.

20. Bronskill SE, Maclagan LC, Walker JD, et al. Trajectories of health system use and survival for community-dwelling persons with dementia: a cohort study. BMJ Open 2020;10(7):e037485.

21. Cagnin A, Di Lorenzo R, Marra C, et al. Behavioral and psychological effects of coronavirus disease-19 quarantine in patients with dementia. Front Psychiatry 2020;11:578015.

22. Whiting D, Atee M, Morris T, et al. Effect of COVID-19 on BPSD severity and caregiver distress: trend data from national dementia-specific behavior support

programs in Australia. Alzheimers Dement 2021;17(S12). https://doi.org/10.1002/alz.058454.

23. Simonetti A, Pais C, Jones M, et al. Neuropsychiatric symptoms in elderly with dementia during COVID-19 pandemic: definition, treatment, and future directions. Front Psychiatry 2020;11:579842. https://doi.org/10.3389/fpsyt.2020.579842.

24. Goodman-Casanova JM, Dura-Perez E, Guzman-Parra J, et al. Telehealth home support during COVID-19 confinement for community-dwelling older adults with mild cognitive impairment or mild dementia: survey study. J Med Internet Res 2020;22(5):e19434.

25. Cohen G, Russo MJ, Campos JA, et al. COVID-19 epidemic in Argentina: worsening of behavioral symptoms in elderly subjects with dementia living in the community. Front Psychiatry 2020;11:866. https://doi.org/10.3389/fpsyt.2020.00866.

26. Moretti R, Caruso P, Giuffré M, et al. COVID-19 lockdown effect on not institutionalized patients with dementia and caregivers. Healthcare 2021;9(7):893.

27. Canevelli M, Bruno G, Cesari M. Providing Simultaneous COVID-19–sensitive and dementia-Sensitive care as We Transition from crisis care to Ongoing care. J Am Med Dir Assoc 2020;21(7):968–9.

28. Lara B, Carnes A, Dakterzada F, et al. Neuropsychiatric symptoms and quality of life in Spanish patients with Alzheimer's disease during the COVID-19 lockdown. Eur J Neurol 2020;27(9):1744–7.

29. Carcavilla N, Pozo AS, González B, et al. Needs of dementia family caregivers in Spain during the COVID-19 pandemic. J Alzheimers Dis JAD 2021;80(2):533–7.

30. Pongan E, Dorey JM, Borg C, et al. COVID-19: association between increase of behavioral and psychological symptoms of dementia during lockdown and caregivers' poor mental health. :9.

31. Tsapanou A, Papatriantafyllou JD, Yiannopoulou K, et al. The impact of COVID-19 pandemic on people with mild cognitive impairment/dementia and on their caregivers. Int J Geriatr Psychiatry 2021;36(4):583–7.

32. Canevelli M, Valletta M, Toccaceli Blasi M, et al. Facing dementia during the COVID -19 outbreak. J Am Geriatr Soc 2020;68(8):1673–6.

33. Borges-Machado F, Barros D, Ribeiro Ó, et al. The effects of COVID-19 home confinement in dementia care: physical and cognitive decline, severe neuropsychiatric symptoms and increased caregiving burden. Am J Alzheimers Dis Dementiasr 2020;35. https://doi.org/10.1177/1533317520976720. 153331752097672.

34. Capozzo R, Zoccolella S, Frisullo ME, et al. Telemedicine for delivery of care in frontotemporal lobar Degeneration during COVID-19 pandemic: results from Southern Italy. J Alzheimers Dis JAD 2020;76(2):481–9.

35. Ali Awan H, Najmuddin Diwan M, Aamir A, et al. SARS-CoV-2 and the brain: what do we know about the causality of 'cognitive COVID? J Clin Med 2021;10(15):3441.

36. Ghaffari M, Ansari H, Beladimoghadam N, et al. Neurological features and outcome in COVID-19: dementia can predict severe disease. J Neurovirol 2021;27(1):86–93.

37. AboJabel H, Idilbi N, Werner P. Hospital staff members' preferences about who should be prioritized to receive the COVID-19 vaccine: people with or without Alzheimer's disease? J Aging Stud 2021;59:100982. https://doi.org/10.1016/j.jaging.2021.100982.

38. Karlsson LC, Soveri A, Lewandowsky S, et al. Fearing the disease or the vaccine: the case of COVID-19. Personal Individ Differ 2021;172:110590. https://doi.org/10.1016/j.paid.2020.110590.

39. Brown EE, Kumar S, Rajji TK, et al. Anticipating and mitigating the impact of the COVID-19 pandemic on Alzheimer's disease and related dementias. Am J Geriatr Psychiatry 2020;28(7):712–21.

40. Cuffaro L, Di Lorenzo F, Bonavita S, et al. Dementia care and COVID-19 pandemic: a necessary digital revolution. Neurol Sci 2020;41(8):1977–9.

41. Dellazizzo L, Léveillé N, Landry C, et al. Systematic review on the mental health and treatment impacts of COVID-19 on neurocognitive disorders. J Pers Med 2021;11(8):746.

42. Sachdev PS, Blacker D, Blazer DG, et al. Classifying neurocognitive disorders: the DSM-5 approach. Nat Rev Neurol 2014;10(11):634–42.

43. WHO. World Health Organization 'Dementia'. 2021. Available at: https://www.who.int/news-room/fact-sheets/detail/dementia. Accessed January 19, 2022.

44. Gauthier S, Cummings J, Ballard C, et al. Management of behavioral problems in Alzheimer's disease. Int Psychogeriatr 2010;22(3):346–72.

45. Kales HC, Gitlin LN, Lyketsos CG. Assessment and management of behavioral and psychological symptoms of dementia. BMJ 2015;350(mar02 7):h369.

46. Tremont G. Family caregiving in dementia. Med Health R 2011;94(2):36–8.

47. Pinquart M, Sörensen S. Differences between caregivers and noncaregivers in psychological health and physical health: a meta-analysis. Psychol Aging 2003; 18(2):250–67.

48. Sallim AB, Sayampanathan AA, Cuttilan A, et al. Prevalence of mental health disorders among caregivers of patients with Alzheimer disease. J Am Med Dir Assoc 2015;16(12):1034–41.

49. Eska K, Graessel E, Donath C, et al. Predictors of institutionalization of dementia patients in mild and moderate stages: a 4-year prospective analysis. Dement Geriatr Cogn Disord Extra 2013;3(1):426–45.

50. Liu K, Chen Y, Lin R, et al. Clinical features of COVID-19 in elderly patients: a comparison with young and middle-aged patients. J Infect 2020;80(6):e14–8.

51. Qian M, Jiang J. COVID-19 and social distancing. J Public Health 2022;30(1): 259–61.

52. Moletta L, Pierobon ES, Capovilla G, et al. International guidelines and recommendations for surgery during Covid-19 pandemic: a systematic review. Int J Surg 2020;79:180–8.

53. Wong BPS, Kwok TCY, Chui KCM, et al. The impact of dementia daycare service cessation due to COVID-19 pandemic. Int J Geriatr Psychiatry 2021;37(1). https://doi.org/10.1002/gps.5621.

54. Giebel C, Cannon J, Hanna K, et al. Impact of COVID-19 related social support service closures on people with dementia and unpaid carers: a qualitative study. Aging Ment Health 2021;25(7):1281–8.

55. Giebel C, Pulford D, Cooper C, et al. COVID-19-related social support service closures and mental well-being in older adults and those affected by dementia: a UK longitudinal survey. BMJ Open 2021;11(1):e045889.

56. yin Lai FH, hung Yan EW, Yu KKying, et al. The protective impact of telemedicine on persons with dementia and their caregivers during the COVID-19 pandemic. Am J Geriatr Psychiatry 2020;28(11):1175–84.

57. Pfefferbaum B, North CS. Mental health and the covid-19 pandemic. N Engl J Med 2020;383(6):510–2.

58. Stockwell S, Trott M, Tully M, et al. Changes in physical activity and sedentary behaviours from before to during the COVID-19 pandemic lockdown: a systematic review. BMJ Open Sport Exerc Med 2021;7(1):e000960.

59. Budnick A, Hering C, Eggert S, et al. Informal caregivers during the COVID-19 pandemic perceive additional burden: findings from an ad-hoc survey in Germany. BMC Health Serv Res 2021;21(1):353.

60. Rainero I, Bruni AC, Marra C, et al. The impact of COVID-19 quarantine on patients with dementia and family caregivers: a nation-wide survey. Front Aging Neurosci 2021;12:625781. https://doi.org/10.3389/fnagi.2020.625781.

61. Cohen G, Russo MJ, Campos JA, et al. Living with dementia: increased level of caregiver stress in times of COVID-19. Int Psychogeriatr 2020;32(11):1377–81.

62. Barguilla A, Fernández-Lebrero A, Estragués-Gázquez I, et al. Effects of COVID-19 pandemic confinement in patients with cognitive impairment. Front Neurol 2020;11:589901. https://doi.org/10.3389/fneur.2020.589901.

63. Hwang Y, Connell LM, Rajpara AR, et al. Impact of COVID-19 on dementia caregivers and factors associated with their anxiety symptoms. Am J Alzheimers Dis Dementiasr 2021;36. https://doi.org/10.1177/15333175211008768. 153331752110087.

64. Altieri M, Santangelo G. The psychological impact of COVID-19 pandemic and lockdown on caregivers of people with dementia. Am J Geriatr Psychiatry 2021; 29(1):27–34.

65. Azevedo LVDS, Calandri IL, Slachevsky A, et al. Impact of social isolation on people with dementia and their family caregivers. J Alzheimers Dis 2021; 81(2):607–17.

66. Ercoli LM, Gammada EZ, Niles P. Coping with dementia caregiving stress and burden during COVID-19. Gerontol Geriatr Res 2021;7 1047.

67. Cousins E, de Vries K, Dening KH. Ethical care during COVID-19 for care home residents with dementia. Nurs Ethics 2021;28(1):46–57.

68. Izcovich A, Ragusa MA, Tortosa F, et al. Prognostic factors for severity and mortality in patients infected with COVID-19: a systematic review. In: Lazzeri C, editor. PLOS ONE 2020;15(11):e0241955.

69. Cox C. Older adults and covid 19: social justice, disparities, and social work practice. J Gerontol Soc Work 2020;63(6–7):611–24.

70. Cipriani G, Di Fiorino M, Cammisuli DM. Dementia in the era of COVID -19. Some considerations and ethical issues. Psychogeriatrics 2022;22(1):132–6.

71. Seminara Donna, Szerszen Anita, Maese John R, et al. Medical home visit programs during COVID-19 state of emergency. Am J Manag Care 2020;26(11): 465–6.

72. Bolt SR, van der Steen JT, Mujezinović I, et al. Practical nursing recommendations for palliative care for people with dementia living in long-term care facilities during the COVID-19 pandemic: a rapid scoping review. Int J Nurs Stud 2021; 113:103781. https://doi.org/10.1016/j.ijnurstu.2020.103781.

73. Iaboni A, Cockburn A, Marcil M, et al. Achieving safe, effective, and compassionate quarantine or isolation of older adults with dementia in nursing homes. Am J Geriatr Psychiatry 2020;28(8):835–8.

74. Liddell K, Ruck Keene A, Holland A, et al. Isolating residents including wandering residents in care and group homes: medical ethics and English law in the context of Covid-19. Int J L Psychiatry 2021;74:101649. https://doi.org/10. 1016/j.ijlp.2020.101649.

75. Weiss EF, Malik R, Santos T, et al. Telehealth for the cognitively impaired older adult and their caregivers: lessons from a coordinated approach. Neurodegener Dis Manag 2021;11(1):83–9.

76. Geddes MR, O'Connell ME, Fisk JD, et al. Remote cognitive and behavioral assessment: report of the Alzheimer Society of Canada Task Force on dementia care best practices for COVID-19. Alzheimers Dement Diagn Assess Dis Monit 2020;12(1). https://doi.org/10.1002/dad2.12111.

77. Tahira AC, Verjovski-Almeida S, Ferreira ST. Dementia is an age-independent risk factor for severity and death in COVID-19 inpatients. Alzheimers Dement 2021;17(11):1818–31.

78. Harrison SL, Fazio-Eynullayeva E, Lane DA, et al. Comorbidities associated with mortality in 31,461 adults with COVID-19 in the United States: a federated electronic medical record analysis. Kretzschmar MEE. PLOS Med 2020;17(9): e1003321. https://doi.org/10.1371/journal.pmed.1003321.

79. Emmerton D, Abdelhafiz AH. Care for older people with dementia during COVID-19 pandemic. SN Compr Clin Med 2021;3(2):437–43. https://doi.org/10.1007/s42399-020-00715-0.

80. Lasa C, Brown EE, Colman R, et al. Invited letter: integrated palliative care in a geriatric mental health setting during the COVID-19 pandemic. Int J Geriatr Psychiatry 2022;37(1). https://doi.org/10.1002/gps.5654. gps.5654.

81. Ting R, Edmonds P, Higginson IJ, et al. Palliative care for patients with severe covid-19. BMJ 2020;m2710. https://doi.org/10.1136/bmj.m2710.

82. Lovell N, Maddocks M, Etkind SN, et al. Characteristics, symptom management, and outcomes of 101 patients with COVID-19 referred for hospital palliative care. J Pain Symptom Manage 2020;60(1):e77–81.

83. Kaasalainen S, Mccleary L, Vellani S, et al. Improving end-of-life care for people with dementia in LTC homes during the COVID-19 pandemic and beyond. Can Geriatr J 2021;24(3):164–9.

84. European Team Eurosurveillanc. Updated rapid risk assessment from ECDC on the novel coronavirus disease 2019 (COVID-19) pandemic: increased transmission in the EU/EEA and the UK. Eurosurveillance 25. 2020.

85. Hsu AT, Lane N, Sinha SK, et al. Understanding the impact of COVID-19 on residents of Canada's long-term care homes – ongoing challenges and policy responses. :19.

86. Burton JK, Bayne G, Evans C, et al. Evolution and effects of COVID-19 outbreaks in care homes: a population analysis in 189 care homes in one geographical region of the UK. Lancet Healthy Longev 2020;1(1):e21–31.

87. McMichael TM, Currie DW, Clark S, et al. Epidemiology of covid-19 in a long-term care facility in king county, Washington. N Engl J Med 2020;382(21): 2005–11.

88. Trabucchi M, De Leo D. Nursing homes or besieged castles: COVID-19 in northern Italy. Lancet Psychiatry 2020;7(5):387–8.

89. Palumbo MV, Rambur B, McKenna LP. Living at home with dementia Now more complicated with COVID-19. Health Soc Work 2021;45(4):289–92.

90. Matias-Guiu JA, Pytel V, Guiu JM. Death rate due to COVID-19 in Alzheimer's disease and frontotemporal dementia. J Alzheimer's Dis 2020;78:537–41.

91. Leontjevas R, Knippenberg IAH, Smalbrugge M, et al. Challenging behavior of nursing home residents during COVID-19 measures in The Netherlands. Aging Ment Health 2021;25(7):1314–9.

92. Lapid MI, Koopmans R, Sampson EL, et al. Providing quality end-of-life care to older people in the era of COVID-19: perspectives from five countries. Int Psychogeriatr 2020;32(11):1345–52.

93. Velayudhan L, Aarsland D, Ballard C. Mental health of people living with dementia in care homes during COVID-19 pandemic. Int Psychogeriatr 2020;32(10): 1253–4.

94. Nussbaumer-Streit B, Mayr V, Dobrescu AI, et al. Quarantine alone or in combination with other public health measures to control COVID-19: a rapid review. Cochrane Infectious Diseases Group, ed. Cochrane Database Syst Rev. 2020. doi:10.1002/14651858.CD013574.

95. Wammes JD, Kolk MSc D, van den Besselaar, et al. Evaluating perspectives of relatives of nursing home residents on the nursing home visiting restrictions during the COVID-19 crisis: a Dutch cross-sectional survey study. J Am Med Dir Assoc 2020;21(12):1746–50.e3.

96. Gordon AL, Goodman C, Achterberg W, et al. Commentary: COVID in care homes—challenges and dilemmas in healthcare delivery. Age Ageing 2020; 49(5):701–5.

97. ter Brugge BPH, van Atteveld VA, Fleuren N, et al. Advance care planning in Dutch nursing homes during the first wave of the COVID-19 pandemic. J Am Med Dir Assoc 2022;23(1):1–6.e1.

98. Olson NL, Albensi BC. Dementia-friendly "design": impact on COVID-19 death rates in long-term care facilities around the world. J Alzheimers Dis 2021;81(2): 427–50.

99. Inzitari M, Risco E, Cesari M, et al. Nursing homes and long term care after COVID-19: a new ERA? J Nutr Health Aging 2020;24(10):1042–6.

100. Werner RM, Hoffman AK, Coe NB. Long-term care Policy after covid-19 — Solving the nursing home crisis. N Engl J Med 2020;383(10):903–5.

101. Kane RL. Assuring quality in nursing home care. J Am Geriatr Soc 1998;46(2): 232–7.

102. Newbould L, Mountain G, Hawley MS, et al. Videoconferencing for health care Provision for older adults in care homes: a review of the research evidence. Int J Telemed Appl 2017;2017:1–7. https://doi.org/10.1155/2017/5785613.

103. Eze ND, Mateus C, Cravo Oliveira Hashiguchi T. Telemedicine in the OECD: an umbrella review of clinical and cost-effectiveness, patient experience and implementation. In: Carter HE, editor. PLOS ONE 2020;15(8):e0237585. https://doi.org/10.1371/journal.pone.0237585.

104. Levere M, Rowan P, Wysocki A. The adverse effects of the COVID-19 pandemic on nursing home resident well-being. J Am Med Dir Assoc 2021;22(5): 948–54.e2.

105. Ryoo N, Pyun JM, Baek MJ, et al. Coping with dementia in the middle of the COVID-19 pandemic. J Korean Med Sci 2020;35(42):e383.

106. Jackson LA, Anderson EJ, Rouphael NG, et al. An mRNA vaccine against SARS-CoV-2 — Preliminary report. N Engl J Med 2020;383(20):1920–31.

107. Walsh EE, Frenck RW, Falsey AR, et al. Safety and Immunogenicity of Two RNA-based covid-19 vaccine Candidates. N Engl J Med 2020;383(25):2439–50.

108. Coronavirus. activity kits, exercise videos rolled out for adults with special needs. The Straits Times (Online). Available at: www.straitstimes.com/singapore/activity-kits-exercise-videos-rolled-out-for-adults-with-specialneeds. Accessed January 19, 2022.

109. Alzheimer's disease association. ADA memo (online). Available at: www.alz.org.sg/adamemo/.

The Impact of the COVID-19 Pandemic on Physical Activity, Function, and Quality of Life

Catherine M. Said, B App Sci (Physio), PhD[a,b,c],
Frances Batchelor, B App Sci, GradDipEd, MHS, PhD[a,d,e],
Gustavo Duque, MD, PhD[c,f],*

KEYWORDS

- COVID-19 • Older persons • Exercise • Physical activity • Quality of life

KEY POINTS

- Older persons diagnosed with COVID-19 have sustained biopsychosocial problems that affect their function, independence, and quality of life.
- Physical activity may reduce the impact of COVID-19 on older people.
- It is essential that communities and governments consider policies and strategies that support older people to become physically active, particularly after recovering from COVID-19.

INTRODUCTION

It is now more than 2 years since the beginning of the COVID-19 pandemic, which has affected people around the globe. The pandemic has directly affected the lives of the many people who contracted COVID-19; nearly 6 million people have lost their lives,[1] and many of those who survive will have symptoms that persist after the initial infection.[2–4] Although the demographics of people infected and the severity of infections have changed over time, older people remain at the highest risk of severe disease. There has also been a substantial indirect impact on people's lives. Many countries imposed restrictions to reduce the spread of infection, including lockdowns and social

[a] Department of Physiotherapy, The University of Melbourne, Melbourne, Victoria, Australia; [b] Department of Physiotherapy, Western Health, Australia; [c] Australian Institute for Musculoskeletal Science (AIMSS), The University of Melbourne and Western Health, St. Albans, Victoria, Australia; [d] National Ageing Research Institute (NARI), Parkville, Australia; [e] School of Nursing and Midwifery, Deakin University, Burwood, Victoria, Australia; [f] Department of Medicine-Western Health, The University of Melbourne, St. Albans, Victoria, Australia
* Corresponding author. Australian Institute for Musculoskeletal Science (AIMSS), Sunshine Hospital, 176 Furlong Road, St. Albans 3021, Victoria, Australia.
E-mail address: gustavo.duque@unimelb.edu.au

Clin Geriatr Med 38 (2022) 519–531
https://doi.org/10.1016/j.cger.2022.04.003
0749-0690/22/© 2022 Elsevier Inc. All rights reserved.

distancing protocols, and mask mandates were common. This article focuses on the impact of the COVID-19 pandemic on physical activity in older people and subsequent effects and implications for function and quality of life.

WHY IS PHYSICAL ACTIVITY IMPORTANT FOR OLDER PEOPLE?

There is overwhelming evidence that physical activity and exercise are critical to the health and well-being of older people. Physical activity, including exercise, is linked with functional abilities, including mobility and independence in personal and community activities of daily living, particularly in older people.[5–9] Reductions in functional ability and mobility are often a precursor to reduced independence and quality of life, institutionalization, and mortality. There is strong evidence that balance and strength exercises reduce the risk of falls by approximately 25%[8,9] and improve function, particularly in older people who are frail or have limited mobility.[7] Recent guidelines from the World Health Organization recognize the importance of physical activity for all older people, including those with chronic health conditions and disabilities.[10,11] It is *strongly recommended* that older adults over the age of 65 years should do at least 150 to 300 minutes of moderate intensity (or an equivalent combination of moderate and vigorous intensity physical activity) every week and that they should include functional balance and strength training 3 days a week to improve function and reduce falls risk. The new guidelines also highlight that even if older people do not meet the guidelines *some physical activity is better than none.* Older people with health conditions and disabilities should be as active as their condition, and abilities allow and should consult with physical activity specialists or health care professionals for advice. Physical activity is critical to maximizing health, well-being, and independence in all older people and vital to minimizing institutionalization.

Physical activity may also reduce the impact of COVID-19 in older people. There is some evidence that regular physical activity improves the immune response.[12–14] A systematic review identified that higher levels of habitual physical activity was associated with a 31% reduction in community-acquired infections (hazard ratio 0.69, 95% confidence interval [CI] 0.61–0.78, 6 studies, N = 557,487 individuals) and 27% reduction in infection-related mortality (hazard ratio 0.64, 95% CI 0.59–0.70, 4 studies, N = 422,813 individuals), although the review did not include any studies specifically investigating the response to COVID-19.[15] Habitual physical activity was also associated with improvement in antibody responses,[15] particularly after vaccination, which are enhanced not only by the immune but also the musculoskeletal system **(Fig. 1)**.[16] An exploration of associations between physical activity at the community level and COVID-19 in the United States found a negative association between physical activity rates at the county level and COVID-19 cases and deaths,[17] after controlling for several variables linked with overall health and COVID-19 risks and mortality, including personal demographics, health rating, employment status, income, insurance status, and rural status. The investigators acknowledge that physical activity may be an indicator of other factors that affect health behaviors and COVID-19 outcomes, such as mask-wearing. Nonetheless, the results of this study provide some evidence that communities that are more physically active have better outcomes from COVID-19. A Canadian study of 24,114 middle-aged and older adults found that low physical activity and high nutritional risk prepandemic were associated with increased odds of reporting a decline in mobility and physical function after confirmed or probable COVID-19 infection[18]; this provides further evidence that older people who are habitually physically active have better outcomes if infected with COVID-19. Because we are likely to continue to see new variants of COVID-19 and the

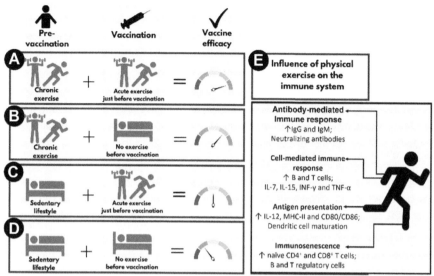

Fig. 1. How acute and chronic physical exercise could interfere with immune system and vaccine efficacy, based on published studies. (A) Subjects who exercise regularly and performed acute exercise just before vaccination; (B) subjects who exercise regularly and did not perform acute exercise just before vaccination; (C) subjects with a sedentary lifestyle who performed acute exercise just before vaccination; (D) subjects with a sedentary lifestyle who did not perform acute exercise just before vaccination. (E) List of main influences of physical exercise on the immune system. Prevaccination is defined as days or months before vaccination; vaccination is defined as the moment of injection; chronic exercise is defined as a regular physical exercise in months or years; acute exercise is defined as moderate/vigorous physical exercise a few minutes or hours before vaccination. (*From* Bortolini MJS, Petriz B, Mineo JR, Resende RO. Why Physical Activity Should Be Considered in Clinical Trials for COVID-19 Vaccines: A Focus on Risk Groups. Int J Environ Res Public Health. 2022;19(3):1853. Published 2022 Feb 7. https://doi.org/10.3390/ijerph19031853; open access under CC BY 4.0)

long-term effectiveness of vaccines is unknown, strategies to increase physical activity in older people must be included in future campaigns to reduce risk and improve outcomes of COVID-19 infection.

PHYSICAL ACTIVITY IN OLDER PEOPLE INFECTED WITH COVID-19

Undoubtedly, the group of people most affected by COVID-19 are those who contracted it. It is currently estimated that more than 440 million people globally have been infected with COVID-19.[1] An unprecedented number of people infected with COVID-19 have required management in intensive care units (ICU) and are at risk for developing postintensive care syndrome (PICS).[19,20] Furthermore, it is recognized that many people diagnosed with COVID-19 have sustained biopsychosocial problems, recognized by the World Health Organization as postacute COVID-19 condition (PACC).[21] Both these groups will have a range of issues that will affect physical activity in both the long and short term.

It is well recognized that survivors of prolonged stays in ICU can experience ongoing morbidity and disability and reduced quality of life, irrespective of their primary admission diagnosis. PICS encompasses physical, psychological, and cognitive domains and includes new or worsening neuromuscular weakness, reduced independence in activities of daily living, anxiety, depression, posttraumatic stress disorder, and cognitive dysfunction,[22] and the risks for developing PICS increase with increasing age.[23] Emerging evidence indicates that people with COVID-19 who require ICU admission are at high risk of developing PICS.[19,20] It is increasingly recognized that this cohort is likely to require ongoing multidisciplinary rehabilitation, including specialized exercise prescription, to optimize function and maximize long-term health outcomes.[24]

Even people who do not require admission to intensive care can have substantial long-term problems post-COVID. PACC is a multisystem disorder that affects function and quality of life. Common features include cough, shortness of breath, headache, fatigue, chest pain, joint pain, depression, and insomnia[25]; however, a recent systematic review identified 55 distinct long-term suboptimal health outcomes for people with COVID-19.[26] There is evidence that even people who do not require hospitalization may have deficits in mobility and physical function. A large study of 24,114 middle-aged and older adults found those who had confirmed or probable COVID-19 (93.3% not hospitalized) had nearly double the odds of reporting a decline in mobility and physical function, compared with people who had not had COVID-19.[18] Although there is currently limited evidence for the management of PACC, there is increasing international recognition that rehabilitation, including specialized exercise prescription, is likely to be a key component of care for this condition.[24,27-29]

There are some key challenges around prescribing exercise and physical activity to people post-COVID-19 infection, particularly those with more severe disease. Some of the complications of COVID-19 include cardiac and autonomic dysfunction and desaturation on exercise. Muscle weakness seems to be common in people with severe COVID-19 infections. It is beyond the scope of this article to provide detailed guidance on exercise and physical activity for this population; however, readers are advised to refer to the many excellent reviews and guidelines in this area (eg, [30-32]). Although little is known about the impact of COVID-19 infection on physical activity in older people, it is likely to be reduced. A survey of physical activity in younger people (younger than 56 years) recovering from COVID-19 found self-reported walking time remained less than pre-COVID levels at both 3 and 6 months, although it should be noted that there are limitations with self-reported physical activity.[33] Nonetheless, clinicians should assess physical activity and function in all older people diagnosed with COVID-19. Performance-based measures, such as the Short Physical Performance Battery or Timed Up and Go, can be administered quickly. However, if these tests cannot be administered, questioning about ability to perform functional tasks such as getting up from a chair, walking up a flight of stairs, concerns regarding balance, or walking several blocks outdoors should be conducted. Referral to exercise specialists should be considered if any persistent reduction in physical activity or function is observed.

PHYSICAL ACTIVITY IN OLDER PEOPLE NOT INFECTED WITH COVID-19

It is now well documented that there have been multiple negative sequelae because of the lockdown restrictions and social distancing requirements necessitated to reduce the spread of COVID-19. Delays in accessing health care for both acute and chronic problems are well documented worldwide.[34] These restrictions have also affected physical activity levels, both via limiting participation in structured exercise and physical activities such as exercise classes, golf, and bowls and via limiting social activities, thus limiting incidental exercise. A systematic review of 25 studies that examined physical activity levels in people older than 60 years found a significant reduction in physical activity during periods of restriction during the pandemic.[35] Although there are limitations with this review, as many studies relied on questionnaires, studies using objective measures such as accelerometry reported reduced step count. The review also noted that reductions in physical activity were greater in countries with more stringent restrictions, whereas studies conducted in countries such as Sweden, which had fewer government-imposed restrictions, did not demonstrate reductions in activity. Furthermore, reduction in physical activity during periods of restriction has also been noted in people with disabilities and chronic conditions[13,36] and people with dementia.[37] Increases in sedentary lifestyle have also been reported.[35,38]

Although consequences of reduced physical activity and increasing sedentary lifestyle may not manifest for some time, there will undoubtedly be an impact on health and function in older people. A systemic review identified a decline in physical fitness of older adults has been observed.[35] A systematic review on the detraining effects after cessation of balance and fall prevention interventions showed a reduction in balance outcomes 4 to 8 weeks after training ceased.[39] Although the review conclusions are limited by the small number of studies included (n = 9), findings indicate older people may be at increased fall risk postpandemic. Several studies have demonstrated links between physical activity, mental health, quality of life, and well-being during the pandemic.[38,40,41] Although these studies do not necessarily prove causation, people who had higher physical activity levels reported better mental health.

Masks may have also affected the amount and types of activities people participated in, particularly older people. Although there is limited evidence on the relationship between masks and activities specifically in older people, a systematic review of 22 studies (n = 1573 participants, mean age 35.6 years ± 15.2 years) found that although masks did not affect exercise performance, masks did increase ratings of perceived exertion and dyspnea and led to slight increases in end tidal CO_2 and heart rate. Although the impact of mask-wearing on exercise performance in older people and those with chronic conditions is not known, it is possible that increases in perceived exertion and dyspnea lead to reduced intensity or duration of physical activity. In addition, masks limit peripheral vision, particularly the lower visual field.[42,43] This may place older people at increased risk of trips and falls, particularly those with gait or balance impairments or visual impairments such as age-related maculopathy, which increase the reliance on peripheral vision. This may have made some older people feel more hesitant when walking outdoors, particularly on uneven surfaces, also leading to restrictions in physical activity.

Reduced levels of physical activity during the pandemic were also likely in people living in residential care.[44,45] Residential care facilities worldwide imposed strict lockdown procedures to minimize infection risk and protect the most vulnerable people. Residents were often restricted from leaving their facilities and, in some cases, confined to their rooms, staff workload was increased, health care workers deemed "nonessential," and volunteers and caregivers were often prevented from attending. Reduced physical activity, alongside the accompanying social isolation, has undoubtedly had a substantial impact on the health and well-being of this vulnerable population.

PHYSICAL ACTIVITY FOR OLDER PEOPLE AND THE FUTURE

We need to recognize that many older people may have reduced their physical activity over the last 2 years. Older people may also have developed new health conditions or have existing health conditions that may not have been optimally managed. Some older people may have become socially isolated, and mental health issues such as depression or anxiety may have developed or emerged. As a consequence, function and mobility may have reduced in some older people; for older people who were already prefrail or frail, these changes may be catastrophic. It is essential that reductions in function are not simply dismissed as "part of growing old" and that we recognize many changes are preventable and reversible. Although there are many barriers to physical activity in older people, we know that health professional recommendations to be active increase the likelihood of people being physically active. To achieve maximum benefit, physical activity must be sustained over the long term, thus behavior change strategies to support formations of new habits must be incorporated. In addition, as communities and health systems rebuild postpandemic, we must consider how we can best support older people at all levels of function to become physically active and optimize their health, function, and quality of life. A summary of recommendations to support older people become more physically active is provided as Clinical Care Points.

The pandemic resulted in a major disruption in the way older people accessed health care and led to many innovative approaches such as the use of technology. There has been a substantial increase in the uptake of telehealth; although it cannot always replace face-to-face exercise prescription, for many older people, it makes it easier to access appropriate care. People can access care in their own home, and the costs and burden of travel are reduced. Additional benefits of telehealth include increased accessibility to specialist services, increased choice for patients, and improved health literacy and health behaviors.[46] Evidence for the effectiveness of exercise or physical activity interventions delivered via telehealth is evolving rapidly. Care delivered via telehealth shows similar outcomes to traditional pulmonary rehabilitation.[47] Evidence for other groups such as stroke is more limited[48,49]; however, a large number of trials have evaluated the feasibility of using telehealth to deliver exercise, with more underway.[50–54] It is essential that mechanisms to support the delivery of physical activity interventions via telehealth to older people are considered and that the effectiveness of telehealth interventions are rigorously evaluated.

Technology has also been used to provide older people at various levels of function with low-cost, accessible, and scalable options to support exercise and physical activity during periods of lockdown. One of the major challenges during the pandemic was that access to individualized assessment and tailoring physical activity and exercise programs was not available. Several online resources were developed, and existing resources promoted, which provided older adults with a variety of physical activity and exercise options tailored to different levels of function and assisted people to make decisions about which options were appropriate for them.[55,56] The Later Life Training group developed "Make Movement Your Mission," releasing 10- to 15-minute movement "snacks" 3 times a day on Facebook and YouTube, which people could either complete in real time or at a time convenient to them.[57] These videos were developed specifically for older people and included options for people at various functional levels. The BBC in the United Kingdom also released a series of videos with examples of physical activities that older people could perform in their homes. More sophisticated digital options, such as the *StandingTall* program, have been used in clinical trials and have the potential to be scalable.[58–61] The *StandingTall* program is delivered via an app and provides high doses of individually tailored exercise that can be safely progressed over time without supervision. Commercial and bespoke devices such as Wii, Xbox, and so forth have been successfully used to increase physical activity in older people. Increasing access to activity monitors via mobile phones and smartwatches makes it easy for people to monitor daily activity, track progress and set goals, and have been shown to increase physical activity.[62,63] However, although technology has the potential to increase accessibility to physical activity support, inequities remain. The use of technology to support health care is influenced by a range of socioeconomic, personal, and cultural factors.[64,65] Moving forward, we must embrace technology to increase physical activity and exercise options, while exploring avenues to reduce inequities in access and tailoring technological solutions to ensure their applicability for use by older people.

There are also a range of exercise programs available, which older people at various levels of function can complete independently in their home, in hospital, or in residential care following an initial assessment of function. For example, the Otago Exercise Program provides tailored strengthening and balance exercises for older people living in the community and has been shown to reduce falls.[66,67] Various programs that use decision trees to guide selection of an appropriate exercise program have been developed and trialed in community, hospital, and long-term care settings.[44,68] The VIVIF-RAIL program has been designed by experts in physical exercise and frailty and provides a range of exercise programs tailored to specific functional levels.[69] It has been shown to prevent functional decline during hospitalization and improve functional capacity in community-dwelling frail/prefrail older adults with mild cognitive impairment.[70,71] Although these programs require some input from health professionals, they do not require intensive supervision. Chair-based exercise programs may also be an option for when exercise programs cannot be completed in standing; although they may not provide the balance challenge of standing programs, they have been shown to lead to improvements in strength.[72]

It is also essential that communities and governments consider policies and strategies that support older people to become physically active and are applicable to their local context. The World Health Organization has made several specific policy recommendations to increase physical activity.[73] Policies must support clear messaging on the importance of physical activity, creation of environments that support physical activity, and provision of opportunities and services that support people to be physically active. The pandemic saw an unprecedented global public media campaign; during the varying levels of restrictions worldwide, exercise was often recognized as one of the few reasons people were allowed to leave their homes.[74] One of the positive consequences of the pandemic is that cycling and walking infrastructure around the world were expanded as people sought alternatives to public transport systems.[75] Other innovative environmental changes that can support physical activity in older people include the creation of Seniors Exercise Parks, with multimodal exercise equipment specifically designed for the older person to improve balance, strength, and functional movement.[76] However, we know many older people, particularly those with health conditions or disability, will require support from appropriately qualified professionals to maximize physical activity. Mechanisms and funding to ensure equitable access to this support are essential. We must continue to build on the activities and learnings from the pandemic as we consider how best to support older people in communities.

SUMMARY

Physical activity is critical for the health and well-being of older people. The pandemic has resulted in a major disruption to the way our communities and health systems function and deliver care. As we move forward, we must consider how to support older people, whose function has deteriorated due to the pandemic, become physically active and how to better support and engage older people in physical activity in the future.

CLINICS CARE POINTS (BASED ON PHYSICAL ACTIVITY RECOMMENDATIONS FROM WOLD HEALTH ORGANIZATION (REFS. 8,10,73))

Physical activity recommendations for older people
- Adults older than 65 years should do at least 150 to 300 minutes of moderate intensity activity (or an equivalent combination of moderate and vigorous intensity physical activity) each week.
- They should include functional balance and strength training 3 days a week.
- Some physical activity is better than none. Even if someone is unable to meet the physical activity guidelines, they should be encouraged to increase their physical activity.
- Older people with chronic health conditions, a disability, a history of falls, or who have concerns about their balance should consult with an exercise specialist for assessment and a program tailored to their needs.
- Function and physical activity should be assessed in older people diagnosed with COVID-19.
- Health professionals should discuss the benefits of regular physical activity with older people.
- Strategies to support behavior change and habit formation should be used.
- Innovative technologies (including online resources, telehealth, apps, activity trackers) may be helpful for increasing physical activity in older people.
- Communities should consider strategies to increase physical activity that are specific to their local context and minimize inequity.

DISCLOSURE

C.M. Said and F. Batchelor were involved in developing the Safe Exercise at Home Web site. The Web site is freely available, and they do not receive any financial compensation from the Web site.

REFERENCES

1. John Hopkins University & Medicine. Coronavirus Resource Centre. John Hopkins University & Medicine. Available at: https://coronavirus.jhu.edu/. Accessed March 3, 2022.
2. Groff D, Sun A, Ssentongo AE, et al. Short-term and long-term rates of postacute sequelae of SARS-CoV-2 infection: a systematic review. JAMA Netw Open 2021; 4(10):e2128568.
3. Nasserie T, Hittle M, Goodman SN. Assessment of the frequency and variety of persistent symptoms among patients with COVID-19: a systematic review. JAMA Netw Open 2021;4(5):e2111417.
4. Taquet M, Dercon Q, Luciano S, et al. Incidence, co-occurrence, and evolution of long-COVID features: a 6-month retrospective cohort study of 273,618 survivors of COVID-19. PLOS Med 2021;18(9):e1003773.
5. Ekelund U, Tarp J, Steene-Johannessen J, et al. Dose-response associations between accelerometry measured physical activity and sedentary time and all cause mortality: systematic review and harmonised meta-analysis. BMJ 2019; 366:l4570.
6. Liu C-j, Latham N. Progressive resistance strength training for improving physical function in older adults. Cochrane Database Syst Rev 2009;3. https://doi.org/10. 1002/14651858.CD002759.pub2.

7. Roberts CE, Phillips LH, Cooper CL, et al. Effect of different types of physical activity on activities of daily living in older adults: systematic review and meta-analysis. J Aging Phys activity 2017;25(4):653–70.

8. Sherrington C, Fairhall N, Kwok W, et al. Evidence on physical activity and falls prevention for people aged 65+ years: systematic review to inform the WHO guidelines on physical activity and sedentary behaviour. Int J Behav Nutr Phys Activity 2020;17(1):144.

9. Sherrington C, Fairhall NJ, Wallbank GK, et al. Exercise for preventing falls in older people living in the community. Cochrane Database Syst Rev 2019;1. https://doi.org/10.1002/14651858.CD012424.pub2.

10. Bull FC, Al-Ansari SS, Biddle S, et al. World Health Organization 2020 guidelines on physical activity and sedentary behaviour. Br J Sports Med 2020;54(24): 1451–62.

11. Izquierdo M, Merchant RA, Morley JE, et al. International exercise recommendations in older adults (ICFSR): expert consensus guidelines. J Nutr Health Aging 2021;25(7):824–53.

12. da Silveira MP, da Silva Fagundes KK, Bizuti MR, et al. Physical exercise as a tool to help the immune system against COVID-19: an integrative review of the current literature. Clin Exp Med 2021;21(1):15–28.

13. Damiot A, Pinto AJ, Turner JE, et al. Immunological implications of physical inactivity among older adults during the COVID-19 pandemic. Gerontology 2020; 66(5):431–8.

14. Filgueira TO, Castoldi A, Santos LER, et al. The relevance of a physical active lifestyle and physical fitness on immune defense: mitigating disease burden, with focus on COVID-19 consequences. Front Immunol 2021;12:587146.

15. Chastin SFM, Abaraogu U, Bourgois JG, et al. Effects of regular physical activity on the immune system, vaccination and risk of community-acquired infectious disease in the general population: systematic review and meta-analysis. Sports Med 2021;51(8):1673–86.

16. Bortolini MJS, Petriz B, Mineo JR, et al. Why physical activity should be considered in clinical trials for COVID-19 vaccines: a focus on risk groups. Int J Environ Res Public Health 2022;19(3):1853.

17. Cunningham GB. Physical activity and its relationship with COVID-19 cases and deaths: analysis of U.S. counties. J Sport Health Sci 2021;10(5):570–6.

18. Beauchamp MK, Joshi D, McMillan J, et al. Assessment of functional mobility after COVID-19 in adults aged 50 Years or older in the Canadian Longitudinal Study on Aging. JAMA Netw Open 2022;5(1):e2146168.

19. Jaffri A, Jaffri UA. Post-Intensive care syndrome and COVID-19: crisis after a crisis? Heart Lung 2020;49(6):883–4.

20. Smith EMT, Lee ACW, Smith JM, et al. COVID-19 and post-intensive care syndrome: community-based care for ICU survivors. Home Health Care Management Pract 2021;33(2):117–24.

21. World Health Organization. A clinical case definition of post COVID-19 condition by a Delphi consensus. 2021. Available at: WHO/2019-nCoV/Post_COVID-19_condition/Clinical_case_definition/2021.1. Accesssed March 12, 2022.

22. Needham DM, Davidson J, Cohen H, et al. Improving long-term outcomes after discharge from intensive care unit: report from a stakeholders' conference. Crit Care Med 2012;40(2):502–9.

23. Lee M, Kang J, Jeong YJ. Risk factors for post-intensive care syndrome: a systematic review and meta-analysis. Aust Crit Care 2020;33(3):287–94.

24. Goodwin VA, Allan L, Bethel A, et al. Rehabilitation to enable recovery from COVID-19: a rapid systematic review. Physiotherapy 2021;111:4–22.
25. Fernández-de-Las-Peñas C, Palacios-Ceña D, Gómez-Mayordomo V, et al. Prevalence of post-COVID-19 symptoms in hospitalized and non-hospitalized COVID-19 survivors: a systematic review and meta-analysis. Eur J Intern Med 2021;92: 55–70.
26. Lopez-Leon S, Wegman-Ostrosky T, Perelman C, et al. More than 50 long-term effects of COVID-19: a systematic review and meta-analysis. Scientific Rep 2021;11(1):16144.
27. Wittmer VL, Paro FM, Duarte H, et al. Early mobilization and physical exercise in patients with COVID-19: a narrative literature review. Complement Ther Clin Pract 2021;43:101364.
28. Jimeno-Almazán A, Pallarés JG, Buendía-Romero Á, et al. Post-COVID-19 syndrome and the potential benefits of exercise. Int J Environ Res Public Health 2021;18(10). https://doi.org/10.3390/ijerph18105329.
29. Liska D, Andreansky M. Rehabilitation and physical activity for COVID-19 patients in the post infection period. Bratisl Lek Listy 2021;122(5):310–4.
30. Thomas P, Baldwin C, Beach L, et al. Physiotherapy management for COVID-19 in the acute hospital setting and beyond: an update to clinical practice recommendations. J Physiother 2022;68(1):8–25.
31. Wade DT. Rehabilitation after COVID-19: an evidence-based approach. Clin Med (Lond) 2020;20(4):359–65.
32. World Health Organization. Rehabilitation needs of people recovering from COVID-19. 2021. Available at: https://wfot.org/assets/resources/Scientific-brief-Rehabilitation-and-COVID-19.pdf.
33. Delbressine JM, Machado FVC, Goërtz YMJ, et al. The impact of post-COVID-19 syndrome on self-reported physical activity. Int J Environ Res Public Health 2021; 18(11). https://doi.org/10.3390/ijerph18116017.
34. Moynihan R, Sanders S, Michaleff ZA, et al. Impact of COVID-19 pandemic on utilisation of healthcare services: a systematic review. BMJ Open 2021;11(3): e045343.
35. Oliveira MR, Sudati IP, Konzen VM, et al. Covid-19 and the impact on the physical activity level of elderly people: a systematic review. Exp Gerontol 2022;159: 111675.
36. Pérez-Gisbert L, Torres-Sánchez I, Ortiz-Rubio A, et al. Effects of the COVID-19 pandemic on physical activity in chronic diseases: a systematic review and meta-analysis. Int J Environ Res Public Health 2021;18(23). https://doi.org/10.3390/ijerph182312278.
37. Lebrasseur A, Fortin-Bédard N, Lettre J, et al. Impact of the COVID-19 pandemic on older adults: rapid review. JMIR Aging 2021;4(2):e26474.
38. Runacres A, Mackintosh KA, Knight RL, et al. Impact of the COVID-19 pandemic on sedentary time and behaviour in children and adults: a systematic review and meta-analysis. Int J Environ Res Public Health 2021;18(21). https://doi.org/10.3390/ijerph182111286.
39. Modaberi S, Saemi E, Federolf PA, et al. A systematic review on detraining effects after balance and fall prevention interventions. J Clin Med 2021;10(20). https://doi.org/10.3390/jcm10204656.
40. Marconcin P, Werneck AO, Peralta M, et al. The association between physical activity and mental health during the first year of the COVID-19 pandemic: a systematic review. BMC Public Health 2022;22(1):209.

41. O'Brien WJ, Badenhorst CE, Draper N, et al. Physical activity, mental health and well-being during the first COVID-19 containment in New Zealand: a cross-sectional study. Int J Environ Res Public Health 2021;(22):18. https://doi.org/10.3390/ijerph182212036.

42. Callisaya M, Hill K, Hill AM, et al. Face masks and risk of falls - a vision for personalised advice and timing. BMJ: Br Med J 2020;371:m4133.

43. Klatt BN, Anson ER. Navigating through a COVID-19 world: avoiding obstacles. J Neurol Phys Ther 2021;45(1):36–40.

44. Aubertin-Leheudre M, Rolland Y. The importance of physical activity to care for frail older adults during the COVID-19 pandemic. J Am Med Dir Assoc 2020; 21(7):973–6.

45. Thiel A, Altmeier D, Frahsa A, et al. Saving lives through life-threatening measures? The COVID-19 paradox of infection prevention in long-term care facilities. Eur Rev Aging Phys Activity 2021;18(1):11.

46. Fisk M, Livingstone A, Pit SW. Telehealth in the context of COVID-19: changing perspectives in Australia, the United Kingdom, and the United States. J Med Internet Res 2020;22(6):e19264.

47. Cox NS, Dal Corso S, Hansen H, et al. Telerehabilitation for chronic respiratory disease. Cochrane Database Syst Rev 2021;1(1):Cd013040.

48. Laver KE, Adey-Wakeling Z, Crotty M, et al. Telerehabilitation services for stroke. Cochrane Database Syst Rev 2020;1(1):CD010255.

49. Ramage ER, Fini NA, Lynch EA, et al. Look before you leap. Interventions supervised via telehealth involving activities in weightbearing or standing positions for people after stroke. A scoping review. Phys Ther 2021;101(6). https://doi.org/10.1093/ptj/pzab073.

50. Bernocchi P, Giordano A, Pintavalle G, et al. Feasibility and clinical efficacy of a multidisciplinary home-telehealth program to prevent falls in older adults: a randomized controlled trial. J Am Med Dir Assoc 2019;20(3):340–6.

51. Flynn A, Preston E, Dennis S, et al. Home-based exercise monitored with telehealth is feasible and acceptable compared to centre-based exercise in Parkinson's disease: a randomised pilot study. Clin Rehabil 2021;35(5): 728–39.

52. English C, Attia J, Bernhardt J, et al. Secondary prevention of stroke: study protocol for a telehealth-delivered physical activity and diet pilot randomised trial (ENAbLE-pilot). Cerebrovasc Dis 2021;50(5):605–11.

53. Bennell KL, Nelligan R, Dobson F, et al. Effectiveness of an internet-delivered exercise and pain-coping skills training intervention for persons with chronic knee pain: a randomized trial. Ann Intern Med 2017;166(7):453–62.

54. Hinman RS, Kimp AJ, Campbell PK, et al. Technology versus tradition: a non-inferiority trial comparing video to face-to-face consultations with a physiotherapist for people with knee osteoarthritis. Protocol for the PEAK randomised controlled trial. Clinical Trial Protocol. BMC Musculoskelet Disord 2020; 21(1):522.

55. Latham N, Coukell A. Home strong: strength through the years. Available at: www.homestrong.net. Accessed March 4, 2022.

56. Safe Exercise at Home Collaborators. Safe exercise at home. Available at: www.safeexerciseathome.org.au. Accessed March 4, 2022.

57. Later life training: make movement Your Mission. Available at: https://www.laterlifetraining.co.uk/make-movement-your-mission-supporting-people-to-move-throughout-the-covid-19-pandemic/. Accessed March 4, 2022.

58. Delbaere K, Valenzuela T, Lord SR, et al. E-health StandingTall balance exercise for fall prevention in older people: results of a two year randomised controlled trial. BMJ 2021;373:n740.

59. Taylor ME, Todd C, O'Rourke S, et al. Implementation of the StandingTall programme to prevent falls in older people: a process evaluation protocol. BMJ Open 2021;11(7):e048395.

60. Miller KJ, Adair BS, Pearce AJ, et al. Effectiveness and feasibility of virtual reality and gaming system use at home by older adults for enabling physical activity to improve health-related domains: a systematic review. Age and Ageing 2014; 43(2):188–95.

61. Neri SG, Cardoso JR, Cruz L, et al. Do virtual reality games improve mobility skills and balance measurements in community-dwelling older adults? Systematic review and meta-analysis. Clin Rehabil 2017;31(10):1292–304.

62. Laranjo L, Ding D, Heleno B, et al. Do smartphone applications and activity trackers increase physical activity in adults? Systematic review, meta-analysis and metaregression. Br J Sports Med 2021;55(8):422–32.

63. Oliveira J S, Sherrington C, Zheng E RY, et al. Effect of interventions using physical activity trackers on physical activity in people aged 60 years and over: a systematic review and meta-analysis. Br J Sports Med 2020;54(20):1188–94.

64. Crawford A, Serhal E. Digital health equity and COVID-19: the innovation curve cannot reinforce the social gradient of health. J Med Internet Res 2020;22(6): e19361.

65. Mahajan S, Lu Y, Spatz ES, et al. Trends and predictors of use of digital health technology in the United States. Am J Med Jan 2021;134(1):129–34.

66. Chiu H-L, Yeh T-T, Lo Y-T, et al. The effects of the otago exercise programme on actual and perceived balance in older adults: a meta-analysis. PLoS One 2021; 16(8):e0255780.

67. Thomas S, Mackintosh S, Halbert J. Does the 'Otago exercise programme' reduce mortality and falls in older adults?: a systematic review and meta-analysis. Age and Ageing 2010;39(6):681–7.

68. Carvalho LP, Kergoat M-J, Bolduc A, et al. A systematic approach for prescribing posthospitalization home-based physical activity for mobility in older adults: the PATH Study. J Am Med Dir Assoc 2019;20(10):1287–93.

69. Izquierdo M, Rodriguez-Mañas L, Sinclair AJ, et al. What is new in exercise regimes for frail older people — how does the Erasmus Vivifrail Project take us forward? J Nutr Health Aging 2016;20(7):736–7.

70. Casas-Herrero Á, Sáez de Asteasu ML, Antón-Rodrigo I, et al. Effects of Vivifrail multicomponent intervention on functional capacity: a multicentre, randomized controlled trial. J Cachexia Sarcopenia Muscle 2022;13(2):884–93.

71. Martínez-Velilla N, Casas-Herrero A, Zambom-Ferraresi F, et al. Effect of exercise intervention on functional decline in very elderly patients during acute hospitalization: a randomized clinical trial. JAMA Intern Med 2019;179(1):28–36.

72. Klempel N, Blackburn NE, McMullan IL, et al. The effect of chair-based exercise on physical function in older adults: a systematic review and meta-analysis. Int J Environ Res Public Health Feb 16 2021;18(4). https://doi.org/10.3390/ijerph18041902.

73. World Health Organization. Global action plan on physical activity 2018–2030: more active people for a healthier world. 2018. Available at: https://apps.who.int/iris/bitstream/handle/10665/272722/9789241514187-eng.pdf.

74. Levinger P, Hill KD. The impact of mass media campaigns on physical activity participation on a global scale: lessons learned from the COVID-19 pandemic. J Phys Activity Health 2020;17(9):857–8.

75. International Transport Forum. Covid-19 transport brief: Re-spacing our cities for resilience, analysis, factors and figures for transport's response to the coronavirus. 2020. Available at: https://www.itf-oecd.org/sites/default/files/respacing-cities-resilience-covid-19.pdf.

76. Levinger P, Dunn J, Panisset MG, et al. The effect of the ENJOY seniors exercise park physical activity program on falls in older people in the community: a prospective pre-post study design. J Nutr Health Aging 2022. https://doi.org/10.1007/s12603-021-1724-1.

Long COVID-19
The Need for an Interdisciplinary Approach

Isabel Rodriguez-Sanchez, PhD, MD[a],
Leocadio Rodriguez-Mañas, PhD, MD[b,c,]*, Olga Laosa, PhD, MD[b,d]

KEYWORDS

- Long COVID • Sarcopenia • Function • Frailty • Multicomponent exercise
- POSITIVE

KEY POINTS

- Long COVID is defined by the World Health Organization (WHO) as a condition that occurs in individuals with a history of probable or confirmed severe acute respiratory syndrome coronavirus-2 (SARS-CoV-2) infection, usually 3 months from the onset of coronavirus disease 2019 (COVID-19) with symptoms that last for at least 2 months and cannot be explained by an alternative diagnosis.
- The epidemiology and etiopathogenesis are not well known and the available data on long COVID in older people are scarce, which may be because of the different symptoms that this population presents, mainly weakness, confusion, and mood alterations.
- Acute illness, immobilization, lack of physical exercise caused by lockdown and hospitalization, among other things, can result in sarcopenia, leading to worsening functional status in the elderly.
- Early detection of worsening functional status through geriatric comprehensive assessment of old people after acute COVID-19 is essential to provide individualized treatment. Rehabilitation programs based on multicomponent physical activity (Vivifrail) associated with adequate nutrition programs are useful to prevent or improve post–COVID-19 sarcopenia in these patients.
- The use of home remote monitoring system (maintaining and improving the intrinsic capacity involving primary care and caregivers [POSITIVE]) allows clinicians to monitor any worsening of the functional status as well as to prevent, through the prescription of individualized exercise, the development of sarcopenia as a fundamental mechanism in the development of the post–COVID-19 syndrome in the elderly.

[a] Geriatrics Department, Hospital Clínico San Carlos, c/ Profesor Martín Lagos s/n, 28040-Madrid, Spain; [b] Servicio de Geriatría, Hospital Universitario de Getafe, Carretera de Toledo, Km 12.5, 28905-Getafe, Spain; [c] Centro de Investigación Biomédica en Red "Fragilidad y Envejecimiento Saludable" (CIBERFES), Instituto de Salud Carlos III, c/ Sinesio Delgado, 10, 28029-Madrid, Spain; [d] Geriatric Research Group, Biomedical Research Foundation at Hospital Universitario de Getafe, Carretera de Toledo, Km 12.5, 28905-Getafe, Spain
* Corresponding author.
E-mail address: leocadio.rodriguez@salud.madrid.org

Clin Geriatr Med 38 (2022) 533–544
https://doi.org/10.1016/j.cger.2022.03.005
0749-0690/22/© 2022 Elsevier Inc. All rights reserved.

LONG COVID: IS PERSISTENT CORONAVIRUS DISEASE 2019 A REAL ENTITY?

To date, more than 260 million cases of coronavirus disease 2019 (COVID-19) infection have been reported worldwide (World Health Organization [WHO] worldwide dashboard). The pandemic is caused by the severe acute respiratory syndrome coronavirus 2 (SARS-CoV-2). Persistent symptoms after viral infection is not a novel concept because there is evidence of similar effects seen in severe acute respiratory syndrome and Middle East respiratory syndrome.[1] This fact, along with the nonspecificity of much of the symptoms observed in the long term in patients after the acute phase of COVID-19, has raised doubts about the true existence of this syndrome, a controversy that persists. However, there are several bodies of evidence suggesting that it is a true syndrome with relevant consequences for the patients and for health systems.

Although the symptoms of the acute phase of COVID-19 infection are estimated to last 2 weeks for the mildest cases and up to 12 weeks for the most severe cases, this is only indicative, because it is highly dependent on other factors such as age, previous functional status, symptoms, and concomitant diseases.[2] The most frequent symptoms include fatigue, dyspnea, myalgia, weakness, headache, and cognitive blunting. In patients with pre-COVID comorbidity, a worsening of preexisting symptoms has been observed.[3] Around 50% of patients with acute symptomatic COVID-19 infection progress to a phase of persistence for more than 4 weeks of some of the clinical manifestations, the so-called postacute sequelae of COVID-19 (PASC).[4] WHO has developed a clinical case definition of the post–COVID-19 condition by Delphi methodology: a condition that occurs in individuals with a history of probable or confirmed SARS-CoV-2 infection, usually 3 months from the onset of COVID-19, with symptoms that last for at least 2 months and cannot be explained by an alternative diagnosis. Symptoms may be new onset following initial recovery from an acute COVID-19 episode or persist from the initial illness. Symptoms may also fluctuate or relapse over time.[5] Among the hypotheses suggested as to the etiopathogenesis of long COVID is the possible persistence of the virus in the host, causing a latent infection, the inflammatory storm, or the existence of autoantibodies that would act against immunomodulatory proteins. However, the cause is still unknown.

Symptoms of long COVID include fatigue or muscle weakness, malaise, dyspnea, headache, and many other neurocognitive conditions described as cognitive impairment, inability to perform everyday physical tasks, and increased likelihood of developing stress, depression, irritability, insomnia, confusion, or frustration.[6] However, other symptoms, such as cardiac, dermatologic, digestive, and ear, nose, and throat disorders, are possible, which makes it difficult to accurately assess the syndrome, its clinical manifestations, and pathogenic factors. Along with the definition that is discussed in this article, there are some others that establish different time framework or different sets of symptoms.

Its epidemiology remains incompletely understood. The numbers vary from one study to another, depending on methodology, whether outpatient or hospital-initiated surveys are used, structure of follow-up programs, comorbidities, length of hospital stay, and with or without intensive care unit stay, among many other factors of variability. Several North American and European studies report an incidence of long COVID of 30% to 90% at 6 months.[7]

There is increasing published evidence on persistent COVID-19 in the general population. It has been published that patients who have had severe COVID-19 and who have required hospital admission are more likely to have symptoms of persistent COVID-19, especially those who have required oxygen supplementation, treatment with enoxaparin, and with a greater number of symptoms in the acute phase, especially dyspnea, cough, and asthenia.[8] Other studies have found that the risk of developing long COVID syndrome is higher in patients with more than 5 symptoms in the acute phase of the infection, and more frequent in women, in obese patients, and in patients with diabetes.[9,10] In addition, a significant association between the presence of fatigue during the acute phase of infection and azithromycin treatment with long COVID has been published.[8]

LONG COVID IN OLDER PEOPLE: MAIN CHARACTERISTICS

Older people meet several of these clinical characteristics, suggesting that they would have been well represented in the data reports currently available in the literature. However, the available data about long COVID concerning older patients are scarce and inconclusive. Although older people was the segment of the population with a most severe impact (not only death but also clinical severity), it is surprising to see that the reported case series about long COVID show that this condition is affecting mainly middle-aged women,[11] raising the potential of underreporting, which seems to be the case according to the report by Groff and colleagues.[12] In this systematic review, from 50 studies where age is reported, in only 3 of them is the median or mean age 70 to 74 years, with no studies with median/mean ages of 75 years and older. An alternative explanation could be that the clinical manifestations of the syndrome are different from those usually observed in the general population and not well recognized, or that some of the symptoms could be misinterpreted as general consequences of the acute disease or hospitalization in older people (functional deterioration, cognitive impairment/delirium), not directly linked to the infection by SARS-CoV-2.

Some investigators have published a prevalence of about 9% of patients interviewed in a cohort of 279 old patients, being significantly more frequent among patients with severe versus mild to moderate acute disease.[13] Among the most frequent symptoms of long COVID syndrome in older patients are mood disorders, including depression (12.2%), fatigue (8.9%), and anxiety (7.5%), with other symptoms such as cough, dyspnea, myalgia, and loss of smell and taste being less frequent.[13] In another study, after interviewing 165 participants with a mean age of 73 years, it was observed that the most frequent symptom was fatigue (53.1%), but breathlessness (51.5%), joint pain (22.2%), and cough (16.7%) were also highly prevalent.[8] In addition, clinical data in patients with a mean age of 60 years show that more than 5% of body weight can be lost within 2 weeks of acute COVID-19 infection.[14]

FUNCTIONAL CONSEQUENCES OF CORONAVIRUS DISEASE 2019 IN OLDER PEOPLE

Short-term and long-term effects on the musculoskeletal system have been described in older people. Although impairments in other organs and systems, such as the respiratory and cardiovascular systems, can help to explain some of the consequences of COVID-19 in the long term, it seems that the disorders on the musculoskeletal system account for the major part of the functional decline. These consequences come from 3 main areas: the effect of the virus and the disease itself, hospitalization, and confinement.

The risk of both sarcopenia and possible cachexia may be much higher in older patients with infection by SARS-CoV-2[15,16] and could play an important role of vulnerability to the post–COVID-19 functional and physical deterioration.[17] Furthermore, it has been observed that the strength of biceps brachii and quadriceps femoris were lower in post–COVID-19 survivors (69% and 54% of the predicted normal value, respectively).[18] The severity of post–COVID-19 sarcopenia could be explained by different factors such as preexisting health conditions in older adults (eg, biological age, inmunosenescence, and inflammaging), cardiovascular and immunologic status, altered diet (anosmia, ageusia, loss of appetite), physical inactivity, and gut microbiota (**Fig. 1**).[15]

The biological basis of the effect of the infection on muscle mass and function derives from several factors linked to the direct damage produced by the virus in several tissues and systems but also to the effect of the response of the organisms, with a special role of the inflammatory response. Muscle hypoxia, the cytokine storm in the presence of a dysfunctional mitochondria, and electrolyte and metabolic disturbances, exacerbated in the presence of increased sedentarism, nutrient deficits, and low physical activity, prompt the development of an impairment in musculoskeletal performance.[19–21]

Hospitalization because of COVID-19 is the second factor to be considered, having effects not only caused by the hospitalization but also by some components of the pharmacologic treatment (mainly corticosteroids). Taken jointly, they are associated

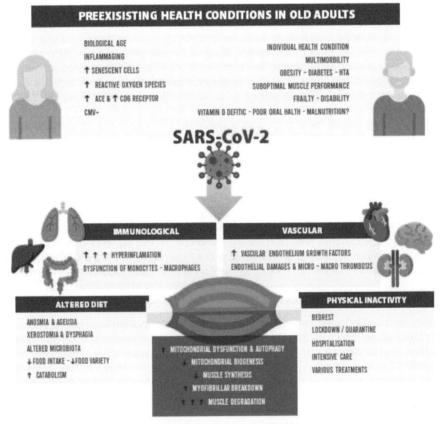

Fig. 1. Physiopathologic pathways of post–COVID-19 sarcopenia. ACE, angiotensin-converting-enzyme; CMV, cytomegalovirus; CD6, cluster of differentiation 6; HTA, Hypertension. (*Adapted from* Piotrowicz, K., Gąsowski, J., Michel, JP. et al. Post-COVID-19 acute sarcopenia: physiopathology and management. Aging Clin Exp Res 33, 2887–2898 (2021). https://doi.org/10.1007/s40520-021-01942-8; under Creative Commons Attribution 4.0 International License.)

with the physiologic outcomes previously mentioned (a reduction in muscle mass and strength, alterations of muscular fiber with a subsequent remodeling of muscle tissue, fatigue, and local systemic inflammation), leading to functional outcomes (accelerated frailty, loss of functional status, chronic disability and dependence) that increase the risk of being discharged to a rehabilitation facility or nursing home, mainly in people more than 80 years old,[22] increasing the health care needs (**Fig. 2**).[23]

The way in which hospitalization because of acute COVID-19 infection contributes to this deleterious outcome of COVID-19 has been studied both in general hospitalization by any cause and in specific hospitalization by COVID-19. Results from the

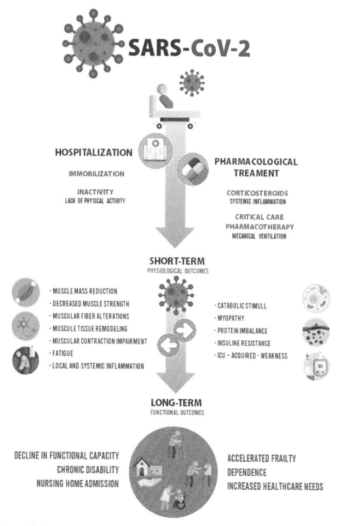

Fig. 2. Effects of pharmacologic treatment and in-hospital immobilization on muscular weakness in old people with COVID-19. (*Adapted from* Sagarra-Romero L, Viñas-Barros A. COVID-19: Short and Long-Term Effects of Hospitalization on Muscular Weakness in the Elderly. Int J Environ Res Public Health. 2020;17(23):8715. Published 2020 Nov 24. https://doi.org/10.3390/ijerph17238715; Open Access under Creative Commons Attribution License.)

Gruppo Lavoro Italiano Sarcopenia-Trattamento e Nutrizione (GLISTEN) study, which could be extrapolated to admission for acute COVID-19 infection, show that there is a 38.4% excess risk of sarcopenia associated with hospital stays of 11 days or more,[24] an usual length in these patients.

Moreover, a recent Norwegian article with a follow-up of 6 months after hospitalization because of COVID-19 has shown a loss of mobility in one-third of the participants, as well as a decreased performance of activities of daily living in 11% of the individuals in the study.[25] In addition, there was the higher risk of persistent functional deterioration, mortality, and readmissions (up to 24-fold, 5-fold, and 4-fold higher, respectively) at 3 months associated with the presence of severe dependence at discharge (Barthel Index <40).[26]

However, this outcome is not restricted to hospitalization in acute care settings. In a recent published study of older people living in long-term care facilities, 29.4% of patients infected by COVID-19 had worsened their previous functional status, even with all physical environmental modifications done for the patients' safety.[27]

The COVID-19 pandemic has led governments to implement unprecedented measures to try to control the spread of the virus. Quarantine, confinement, and social isolation have been widely used measures, especially in the elderly population, where COVID-19 mortality has been higher. Lockdown in older people with and without COVID-19, disregarding its cause, has been related to a large decrease of vigorous and moderate intensity physical activity,[28–33] especially in men,[33] and walking time,[29,30,33] which can accelerate the loss of muscle mass (sarcopenia), increased body fat, and worsening function. According to the WHO recommendations on physical activity, older adults should participate in 150 min/wk of moderate-intensity or 75 min/wk of vigorous-intensity activity.[34] These thresholds not only have not been reached during the COVID-19 quarantine but also sedentary behavior has increased (up to 2 h/d of sitting time),[30,33,35,36] taking into account that confinement and social isolation interrupted not only the spontaneous physical activity but also any supervised exercise program in these older people. As recently published, physical activity was reduced to one-third of baseline, and sedentary time increased from 5 to 8 h/d according to a survey of people older than 55 years during the first wave of the pandemic.[37] Consequently, up to 10% of this population could have developed muscle function loss,[38–40] especially those people who had recovered from SARS-CoV-2 infection,[38,39] accelerating the risk of frailty and sarcopenia.[41,42]

In addition, physical inactivity in older people caused by COVID-19 lockdown has a negative impact on nutrition behavior, with an increased risk to 2- to 4-fold for developing nutritional deficits.[43] Nutritional changes, especially in low-income populations, contribute to worsening sarcopenia and function. Data published in adult and old populations show a reduction in the consumption of vegetables, legumes, and fruits and an increase in the consumption of rice, meat, dairy products, and fast food during the first period of confinement.[44,45] In older people, to be male, social isolation or greater feelings of loneliness, poor housing conditions, as well as a higher prevalence of chronic morbidities are risk factors for developing unhealthier lifestyles or mental health declines during confinement. In contrast, having a good adherence to the Mediterranean diet or doing physical activity before the confinement were protective for the development of unhealthier lifestyles during confinement. It must be highlighted that most of these changes reversed after the end of confinement.[45] The insufficient consumption of essential nutrients for the maintenance of muscle mass, especially amino acids such as leucine, together with the increase in obesity, inflammatory mechanisms characteristic of COVID-19, and the lack of physical activity, could result in sarcopenic obesity.[15] Moreover, these changes in nutritional habits and physical activity may generate changes in gut microbiota, which is known to be related to the severity of COVID-19.[46]

In addition, the role of some of the drugs used in the treatment of acute COVID-19 infection may also act on skeletal muscle, producing sarcopenia in patients with prolonged treatments, in addition to the effect in the acute phase of the disease previously mentioned.

THE GERIATRIC CARE MODEL AND ITS APPLICATION TO THE SPECIFIC CASE OF PERSISTENT CORONAVIRUS DISEASE: COORDINATION OF CARE AND COMPREHENSIVE CARE

As is the usual case in geriatric medicine, functional decline in older people with long COVID should be the cornerstone of the approach to these patients, along with the persistent dyspnea, fatigue, or musculoskeletal pain. In addition, altered diet because of gastrointestinal complaints, anosmia, and dysgeusia could precipitate or impair a sarcopenia condition, leading to a lower functional status, a worsening in instrumental and basic activities of daily living, and a higher risk of falls.[23] In addition, this loss of function could worsen psychological health (depression, anxiety, a lower quality of sleep) and increase the need of social resources (home assistance or new institutionalizations),[22,23] promoting the scenario where an integrated, comprehensive, coordinated, and continued care is needed.

Geriatric medicine has been characterized by a comprehensive care, coordinating the required care of older people according to their needs. Thanks to the information obtained through the geriatric comprehensive assessment and the availability of the different geriatric care levels (outpatient office, rehabilitation unit, geriatric day hospital, institutionalized and noninstitutionalized long-term care), it is possible to provide the best personalized care.

Because the management of the functional decline is the main pillar of the treatment of these patients, promoting self-governance and social participation in the community has a protective effect on physical function, increasing the levels of physical activity.[33–36] The benefits of physical activity are widely known: greater muscle mass; better balance and cognitive function; and lower comorbidities, falls, frailty, sarcopenia, and disability in older people.[22,23,33,34,38–43] In addition, related to SARS-CoV-2, physical activity improves immune function,[47] having a potential protective effect in the older population.

Some programs of functional rehabilitation or telerehabilitation have been proposed, as well as respiratory rehabilitation. First of all, it is important to tailor the multicomponent exercise program not only to the patient but also to where it is going to take place. For older adults who exercise at home, body-weight exercises are crucial, being safe and effective, with chairs, walls, and floor being used to perform them. A Brazilian telerehabilitation program following discharge after COVID-19 stratified the patients according to their Barthel Index to assess different types of physical therapy and time of follow-up. In addition, they also evaluated the need for a nonphysical rehabilitation program: speech-language pathologist for dysphagia, cardiac rehabilitation if oxygen therapy was needed or for worsened dyspnea, occupational therapy if there was fine motor control or cognition decline, physiatrist if pain rated greater than 5, dietitian if weight loss, and psychologist if the patient was anxious or depressed.[48] Other options that have been proved effective in older people at home include the Vivifrail program,[49] which is also useful in older people in nursing homes with COVID-19.[50] Another arm of intervention is pulmonary rehabilitation, showing an improvement of pulmonary function, quality of life, and anxiety levels after a 6-week program.[51–53]

To prevent or improve post–COVID-19 sarcopenia in these patients, it is important to ensure an adequate intake of proteins, vitamins, and minerals, oral nutritional supplements (ONS) being included in the diet, especially when the diet alone may not be sufficient. Thus, the recommendation is to provide at least 400 kcal/d with ONS, with 30 g of protein or more for, at minimum, 30 days.[54] If a high risk of malnutrition exists, these requirements increase up to 600 kcal/d.[55] Although changes in gut microbiota are known to be linked to immune response, and prebiotics and probiotics seem to have a benefit in frail people, the evidence is still unclear in post–COVID-19 older people.[56]

Cognitive consequences related to infection by SARS-CoV-2 may affect physical activity and sarcopenia[57] in long COVID, making cognitive training programs potentially useful.[58,59] A few programs to fight loneliness have been developed, especially in nursing homes. The Telephone Outreach in the COVID-19 Outbreak (TOCO) is a pilot telephone program implemented by medical students of Yale University in which once per week they call older people living in nursing homes. Residents and volunteers share stories of their lives, observing a positive experience.[60]

As mentioned earlier, an increase of social resources is needed as a consequence of higher functional limitations and disability after COVID-19. An early evaluation is important to assess the future needs of the patient, in which the comprehensive geriatric assessment could be helpful, working hand in hand with social workers.

THE ROLE OF TECHNOLOGY IN LONG COVID SYNDROME IN OLD PEOPLE

During the months of confinement and social isolation caused by COVID-19, mobile health (mHealth) and digital health (eHealth) technologies offered a means by which older people could engage in physical activity. However, there was low to moderate evidence that interventions delivered via mHealth or eHealth approaches may be effective in increasing physical activity in older adults in the short term.[61]

POSITIVE (an acronym for maintaining and improving the intrinsic capacity involving primary care and caregivers) technology is a European Union Institute of Innovation and Technology project (EIT-Health–funded project).[62] Its main objective is to make available a home remote monitoring system that allows better management and treatment of frailty, in order to maintain or improve the intrinsic capacity of the elderly, through a telematic platform of services. The home monitoring system consists of a series of questionnaires and 3 sensors that measure variables such as gait speed, power in the lower extremities, and involuntary weight loss. In addition, POSITIVE has a system of personalized prescription of physical exercise based on the Vivifrail program, as well as a nutritional plan and monitoring of functional status.[63] The use of this technology will allow clinicians to monitor any worsening of the functional status as well as to prevent, through the prescription of individualized exercise, the development of sarcopenia as a fundamental mechanism in the development of the symptoms of post–COVID-19 syndrome in older people.

CLINICS CARE POINTS

- A proactive search for long COVID syndrome in older people in the acute phase of the infection is recommended, taking into account the high prevalence and the difficulty of identifying the syndrome in some old patients.
- Functional decline and its consequences should be the focus of attention in the integrated and coordinated care of older people with long COVID syndrome, establishing the level of geriatric care needed for each person, according to the comprehensive geriatric assessment.

- A multicomponent and individualized intervention program should be prescribed, taking into account not only the characteristics of the patient but also the place to do it. Several programs of personalized physical exercise to be performed in different settings of care are accessible. A protein intake of at least 30 g/d should be provided for a minimum of 30 days. The use of prebiotics and probiotics is still controversial.
- A cognitive and social approach should be done to avoid cognitive and mood disorders.
- Technologies currently available in the market can be useful in monitoring the evolution of these patients and in the provision of multicomponent interventions.

FUNDING

CIBER-ISCIII (CB16/10/00464), co-funded by FEDER. A Way to Make Europe.

DISCLOSURE

The authors have nothing to disclose.

REFERENCES

1. Malik P, Patel K, Pinto C, et al. Post-acute COVID-19 syndrome (PCS) and health-related quality of life (HRQoL)-A systematic review and meta-analysis. J Med Virol 2022;94(1):253–62.
2. Landi F, Carfì A, Benvenuto F, et al. Predictive factors for a new positive nasopharyngeal swab among patients recovered from COVID-19. Am J Prev Med 2021; 60(1):13–9.
3. Fernández-de-Las-Peñas C, Florencio LL, Gómez-Mayordomo V, et al. Proposed integrative model for post-COVID symptoms. Diabetes Metab Syndr 2021;15(4): 102159.
4. Greenhalgh T, Knight M, A'Court C, et al. Management of post-acute covid-19 in primary care. BMJ 2020;370:m3026.
5. Douglas H, Georgiou A, Westbrook J. Social participation as an indicator of successful aging: an overview of concepts and their associations with health. Aust Health Rev 2017;41(4):455–62.
6. Jimeno-Almazán A, Pallarés JG, Buendía-Romero Á, et al. Post-COVID-19 syndrome and the potential benefits of exercise. Int J Environ Res Public Health 2021;18(10).
7. Naeije R, Caravita S. Phenotyping long COVID. Eur Respir J 2021;58(2).
8. Tosato M, Carfì A, Martis I, et al. Prevalence and predictors of persistence of COVID-19 symptoms in older adults: a single-center study. J Am Med Dir Assoc 2021;22(9):1840–4.
9. Sudre CH, Murray B, Varsavsky T, et al. Attributes and predictors of long COVID. Nat Med 2021;27(4):626–31.
10. Feldman EL, Savelieff MG, Hayek SS, et al. COVID-19 and diabetes: a collision and collusion of two diseases. Diabetes 2020;69(12):2549–65.
11. Davis HE, Assaf GS, McCorkell L, et al. Characterizing long COVID in an international cohort: 7 months of symptoms and their impact. EClinicalMedicine 2021;38:101019.
12. Groff D, Sun A, Ssentongo AE, et al. Short-term and long-term rates of postacute sequelae of SARS-CoV-2 infection: a systematic review. JAMA Netw Open 2021; 4(10):e2128568.
13. P S, Madhavan S, Pandurangan V. Prevalence, pattern and functional outcome of post COVID-19 syndrome in older adults. Cureus 2021;13(8):e17189.

14. Di Filippo L, De Lorenzo R, D'Amico M, et al. COVID-19 is associated with clinically significant weight loss and risk of malnutrition, independent of hospitalisation: a post-hoc analysis of a prospective cohort study. Clin Nutr 2021;40(4): 2420–6. Edinb Scotl.

15. Piotrowicz K, Gąsowski J, Michel J-P, et al. Post-COVID-19 acute sarcopenia: physiopathology and management. Aging Clin Exp Res 2021;33(10):2887–98.

16. Welch C, Greig C, Masud T, et al. COVID-19 and acute sarcopenia. Aging Dis 2020;11(6):1345–51.

17. Carfì A, Bernabei R, Landi F. Persistent symptoms in patients after acute COVID-19. JAMA 2020;324(6):603–5.

18. Paneroni M, Simonelli C, Saleri M, et al. Muscle strength and physical performance in patients without previous disabilities recovering from COVID-19 pneumonia. Am J Phys Med Rehabil 2021;100(2):105–9.

19. Ayres JS. A metabolic handbook for the COVID-19 pandemic. Nat Metab 2020; 2(7):572–85.

20. Moreno Fernández-Ayala DJ, Navas P, López-Lluch G. Age-related mitochondrial dysfunction as a key factor in COVID-19 disease. Exp Gerontol 2020;142:111147.

21. Kirwan R, McCullough D, Butler T, et al. Sarcopenia during COVID-19 lockdown restrictions: long-term health effects of short-term muscle loss. GeroScience 2020;42(6):1547–78.

22. Herrmann ML, Hahn J-M, Walter-Frank B, et al. COVID-19 in persons aged 70+ in an early affected German district: risk factors, mortality and post-COVID care needs-a retrospective observational study of hospitalized and non-hospitalized patients. PLoS One 2021;16(6):e0253154.

23. Sagarra-Romero L, Viñas-Barros A. COVID-19: short and long-term effects of hospitalization on muscular weakness in the elderly. Int J Environ Res Public Health 2020;23:17.

24. Martone AM, Bianchi L, Abete P, et al. The incidence of sarcopenia among hospitalized older patients: results from the Glisten study. J Cachexia Sarcopenia Muscle 2017;8(6):907–14.

25. Walle-Hansen MM, Ranhoff AH, Mellingsæter M, et al. Health-related quality of life, functional decline, and long-term mortality in older patients following hospitalisation due to COVID-19. BMC Geriatr 2021;21(1):199.

26. Carrillo-Garcia P, Garmendia-Prieto B, Cristofori G, et al. Health status in survivors older than 70 years after hospitalization with COVID-19: observational follow-up study at 3 months. Eur Geriatr Med 2021;12(5):1091–4.

27. Vallecillo G, Anguera M, Martin N, et al. Effectiveness of an acute care for elders unit at a long-term care facility for frail older patients with COVID-19. Geriatr Nurs 2021;42(2):544–7.

28. Sepúlveda-Loyola W, Rodríguez-Sánchez I, Pérez-Rodríguez P, et al. Impact of social isolation due to COVID-19 on health in older people: mental and physical effects and recommendations. J Nutr Health Aging 2020;24(9):938–47.

29. Castañeda-Babarro A, Arbillaga-Etxarri A, Gutiérrez-Santamaría B, et al. Physical Activity Change during COVID-19 Confinement. Int J Environ Res Public Health 2020;17(18):6878.

30. Trabelsi K, Ammar A, Masmoudi L, et al. Sleep quality and physical activity as predictors of mental wellbeing variance in older adults during COVID-19 lockdown: ECLB COVID-19 international online survey. Int J Environ Res Public Health 2021;18(8).

31. Suzuki Y, Maeda N, Hirado D, et al. Physical activity changes and its risk factors among community-dwelling Japanese older adults during the COVID-19

epidemic: associations with subjective well-being and health-related quality of life. Int J Environ Res Public Health 2020;17(18).

32. Okely JA, Corley J, Welstead M, et al. Change in physical activity, sleep quality, and psychosocial variables during COVID-19 lockdown: evidence from the lothian birth cohort 1936. Int J Environ Res Public Health 2020;1:18.

33. Sasaki S, Sato A, Tanabe Y, et al. Associations between socioeconomic status, social participation, and physical activity in older people during the COVID-19 pandemic: a cross-sectional study in a northern Japanese city. Int J Environ Res Public Health 2021;18(4).

34. World Health Organization. Global recommendations on physical activity for health. Geneva Switzerland: WHO Press; 2010.

35. Sañudo B, Fennell C, Sánchez-Oliver AJ. Objectively-assessed physical activity, sedentary behavior, smartphone use.

36. Fernández-García ÁI, Marin-Puyalto J, Gómez-Cabello A, et al. Impact of the home confinement related to COVID-19 on the device-assessed physical activity and sedentary patterns of Spanish older adults. Biomed Res Int 2021;2021: 5528866.

37. Ammar A, Trabelsi K, Brach M, et al. Effects of home confinement on mental health and lifestyle behaviours during the COVID-19 outbreak: insights from the ECLB-COVID19 multicentre study. Biol Sport 2021;38(1):9–21.

38. O'Hara J. Rehabilitation after COVID-19. Mayo Clinic News Network; 2020. Available at.

39. Moro T, Paoli A. When COVID-19 affects muscle: effects of quarantine in older adults. Eur J Transl Myol 2020;30(2):9069.

40. da Rocha AQ, Lobo PCB, Pimentel GD. Muscle function loss and gain of body weight during the COVID-19 pandemic in elderly women: effects of one year of lockdown. J Nutr Health Aging 2021;25(8):1028–9.

41. Hartley P, Costello P, Fenner R, et al. Change in skeletal muscle associated with unplanned hospital admissions in adult patients: a systematic review and meta-analysis. PLoS One 2019;14(1):e0210186.

42. Bell KE, von Allmen MT, Devries MC, et al. Muscle disuse as a pivotal problem in sarcopenia-related muscle loss and dysfunction. J Frailty Aging 2016;5(1):33–41.

43. Visser M, Schaap LA, Wijnhoven HAH. Self-reported impact of the COVID-19 pandemic on nutrition and physical activity behaviour in Dutch older adults living independently. Nutrients 2020;12(12).

44. Sidor A, Rzymski P. Dietary choices and habits during COVID-19 lockdown: experience from Poland. Nutrients 2020;12(6).

45. García-Esquinas E, Ortolá R, Gine-Vázquez I, et al. Changes in health behaviors, mental and physical health among older adults under severe lockdown restrictions during the COVID-19 pandemic in Spain. Int J Environ Res Public Health 2021;18(13).

46. Sarkar A, Harty S, Moeller AH, et al. The gut microbiome as a biomarker of differential susceptibility to SARS-CoV-2. Trends Mol Med 2021;27(12):1115–34.

47. Gjevestad GO, Holven KB, Ulven SM. Effects of exercise on gene expression of inflammatory markers in human peripheral blood cells: a systematic review. Curr Cardiovasc Risk Rep 2015;9(7):34.

48. Leite VF, Rampim DB, Jorge VC, et al. Persistent symptoms and disability after COVID-19 hospitalization: data from a comprehensive telerehabilitation program. Arch Phys Med Rehabil 2021;102(7):1308–16.

49. Romero-García M, López-Rodríguez G, Henao-Morán S, et al. Effect of a multicomponent exercise program (VIVIFRAIL) on functional capacity in elderly

ambulatory: a non-randomized clinical trial in mexican women with dynapenia. J Nutr Health Aging 2021;25(2):148–54.

50. Courel-Ibáñez J, Pallarés JG, García-Conesa S, et al. Supervised exercise (vivif-rail) protects institutionalized older adults against severe functional decline after 14 weeks of COVID confinement. J Am Med Dir Assoc 2021;22(1):217–9.e2.

51. Gautam AP, Arena R, Dixit S, et al. Pulmonary rehabilitation in COVID-19 pandemic era: the need for a revised approach. Respirol Carlton Vic 2020; 25(12):1320–2.

52. Boukhris M, Hillani A, Moroni F, et al. Cardiovascular implications of the COVID-19 pandemic: a global perspective. Can J Cardiol 2020;36(7):1068–80.

53. Liu K, Zhang W, Yang Y, et al. Respiratory rehabilitation in elderly patients with COVID-19: a randomized controlled study. Complement Ther Clin Pract 2020; 39:101166.

54. Barazzoni R, Bischoff SC, Breda J, et al. ESPEN expert statements and practical guidance for nutritional management of individuals with SARS-CoV-2 infection. Clin Nutr Edinb Scotl 2020;39(6):1631–8.

55. Cawood AL, Walters ER, Smith TR, et al. A review of nutrition support guidelines for individuals with or recovering from COVID-19 in the community. Nutrients 2020;12(11).

56. Jayanama K, Theou O. Effects of probiotics and prebiotics on frailty and ageing: a narrative review. Curr Clin Pharmacol 2020;15(3):183–92.

57. Alonso-Lana S, Marquié M, Ruiz A, et al. Cognitive and neuropsychiatric manifestations of COVID-19 and effects on elderly individuals with dementia. Front Aging Neurosci 2020;12:588872.

58. Bernini S, Stasolla F, Panzarasa S, et al. Cognitive telerehabilitation for older adults with neurodegenerative diseases in the COVID-19 era: a perspective study. Front Neurol 2020;11:623933.

59. Salawu A, Green A, Crooks MG, et al. A proposal for multidisciplinary tele-rehabilitation in the assessment and rehabilitation of COVID-19 survivors. Int J Environ Res Public Health 2020;17(13).

60. van Dyck LI, Wilkins KM, Ouellet J, et al. Combating heightened social isolation of nursing home elders: the telephone outreach in the COVID-19 outbreak program. Am J Geriatr Psychiatry 2020;28(9):989–92.

61. McGarrigle L, Todd C. Promotion of physical activity in older people using mhealth and ehealth technologies: rapid review of reviews. J Med Internet Res 2020;22(12):e22201.

62. Barrio Cortes J, Guevara Guevara T, Aguirre Cocha KP, et al. [Positive Project: maintenance and improvement of intrinsic capacity involving primary care and caregivers through a home monitoring system and a telematic services platform. Rev Esp Salud Publica 2021;8:95.

63. Casas-Herrero A, Anton-Rodrigo I, Zambom-Ferraresi F, et al. Effect of a multi-component exercise programme (VIVIFRAIL) on functional capacity in frail community elders with cognitive decline: study protocol for a randomized multicentre control trial. Trials 2019;20(1):362.

The Impact of Long COVID-19 on Muscle Health

Montserrat Montes-Ibarra, MSc[a], Camila L.P. Oliveira, PhD[a], Camila E. Orsso, MSc[a], Francesco Landi, MD[b,c,d,e], Emanuele Marzetti, MD, PhD[e,f,g], Carla M. Prado, PhD, RD[a,*]

KEYWORDS

- COVID-19 • Postacute COVID-19 syndrome • Muscle mass • Aging
- Body composition • Muscle strength • Muscle function • Quality of life

KEY POINTS

- Long COVID negatively impacts muscle mass, function, and quality of life.
- Longitudinal studies, including long-term assessment of muscle mass and function, can help identify the impact of long COVID on muscle health.
- Respiratory muscle dysfunction may be a marker of muscle wasting and recovery outcome during long COVID.
- Age differences should be explored in future studies to better understand how long COVID affects muscle health across the life course.

INTRODUCTION

The World Health Organization (WHO) has recently created a clinical case definition to frame a condition of symptom persistence following a coronavirus disease 2019 (COVID-19).[1] The condition, known as post-COVID-19, postacute sequelae of COVID-19, or long COVID, develops in individuals with a history of probable or

C.M. Prado has received honoraria and/or paid consultancy from Abbott Nutrition, Nutricia, Nestlé Health Science, Fresenius Kabi, and Pfizer. The other authors declare that they have no known conflicts of interest.

[a] Human Nutrition Research Unit, Department of Agricultural, Food, & Nutritional Science, University of Alberta, 113 Street and 87 Avenue NW, 2-004 Li Ka Shing Center for Health Research Innovation, Edmonton, Alberta, Canada; [b] Department of Geriatrics, Neurosciences and Orthopaedics, Catholic University of the Sacred Heart, Rome, Italy; [c] Geriatric Department, Fondazione Policlinico Universitario Agostino Gemelli' IRCCS, Rome, Italy; [d] Department of Translational and Precision Medicine, Sapienza University of Rome, Rome, Italy; [e] Center for Geriatric Medicine (Ce.M.I.), Università Cattolica del Sacro Cuore, L.go F. Vito 1, Rome 00168, Italy; [f] Department of Geriatrics and Orthopedics, Università Cattolica del Sacro Cuore, Rome, Italy; [g] Orthogeriatric Unit, Fondazione Policlinico Universitario "Agostino Gemelli" IRCCS, Rome, Italy
* Corresponding author.
E-mail address: carla.prado@ualberta.ca

confirmed SARS-CoV-2 infection in the past 3 months and encompasses a wide range of signs and symptoms that persists for weeks or months and cannot be explained by an alternative diagnosis. Long COVID symptoms can develop de novo after acute COVID-19 or persist from the initial illness. Common symptoms include, but are not limited to shortness of breath, fatigue, weakness, cognitive dysfunction, body aches, sore throat, cough, diarrhea, anosmia, and dysgeusia.[2,3] It has been estimated that up to 80% of people who recovered from a COVID-19 episode experience at least one long-term symptom.[4,5]

Long COVID has been shown to negatively impact several organs and body systems, including skeletal muscle.[6] This organ is essential for movement, balance, posture, daily activities, and a variety of metabolic functions.[7] Indeed, more than 60% of individuals presenting with long COVID have reported fatigue, lower mobility, and weakness.[8,9] Interestingly, a high prevalence of skeletal muscle weakness and low physical performance has been reported in COVID-19 survivors without prior musculoskeletal problems.[10] Older adults are at increased risk of developing musculoskeletal symptoms during long COVID,[11,12] possibly because of the combined effect of viral infection and preexisting age-related declines in muscle mass and function.

The purpose of this narrative review is to describe the potential long-term effects of COVID-19 on muscle health in adults. We used the term muscle health to describe muscle mass and function (ie, strength and performance). Here, we describe muscle health outcomes in people with long COVID presenting with different degrees of disease severity and assessed by different body composition and physical function methods. In addition, we report the impact of long COVID on quality of life (QoL) related to muscle health.

MECHANISMS OF MUSCLE DAMAGE IN LONG COVID

After entering the human body, the spike protein of SARS-CoV-2 binds to the cell membrane receptor angiotensin converter enzyme 2 (ACE2) using the transmembrane protease, serine 2 (TMPRSS2) to deliver its genetic material.[13,14] Upon cellular entry, the virus replicates and causes disruption of cellular functions, leading to cell death and tissue dysfunction.[15] Because ACE2 and TMPRSS2 are expressed in most tissues and organs, SARS-CoV-2 can invade and cause damage to almost all body systems, including the skeletal muscle.[16] In addition to direct virus-mediated injury, other factors contributing to muscle damage during a COVID-19 episode include systemic inflammation, electrolyte disturbances, critical ill myopathy, drugs (eg, corticosteroids), and hypoxia.[16] Some of these mechanisms and factors are likely to play a role in musculoskeletal damage and its related outcomes in long COVID.

Inflammation is advocated as one of the primary factors associated with muscle catabolism in patients with long COVID.[10] Systemic inflammation sustained by increased blood levels of interferon gamma, C-reactive protein, interleukin (IL) 6, IL-2, IL-10, and tumor necrosis factor α has been described in people with long COVID.[17,18] These proinflammatory cytokines are well known for their ability to negatively impact muscle protein metabolism through triggering catabolic pathways and suppressing anabolism.[19] The mechanisms underlying the transition from acute to chronic inflammation after a COVID-19 episode are largely unknown. Anomalous microclots enriched in acute-phase inflammatory molecules and resistant to fibrinolysis have been found in blood samples of individuals with long COVID.[20] Hence, it is plausible that inflammatory cytokines trapped within microclots may leak into the circulation, thereby maintaining a state of chronic inflammation. SARS-CoV-2 infection was also shown to cause long-term proinflammatory reprogramming of macrophages, possibly via epigenetic modifications.[21] In older COVID-19 survivors, SARS-CoV-2–induced long-term inflammation may superimpose to the age-dependent chronic inflammation (inflamm-aging), leading to more severe disruption of muscle metabolic homeostasis.[5] Over time, proinflammatory cytokines lead to muscle fiber proteolysis, decreased protein synthesis, hindered capacity of satellite cells to proliferate and differentiate, and eventually fibrosis.[15]

Muscular issues in long COVID are more likely to occur in patients with more severe diseases who had been admitted to the intensive care unit (ICU).[22,23] However, Doykov and colleagues[24] observed an increase in proinflammatory biomarkers and disruption of muscle metabolic homeostasis 40 to 60 days after initial diagnosis in individuals who had mild and asymptomatic COVID-19.

Physical inactivity potentially exacerbated by quarantine and hospitalization has also a major impact on muscle mass and function.[6] Lastly, inadequate dietary intake and poor nutritional status, which are common during a COVID-19 episode, negatively impact skeletal muscle during recovery.[25,26] Bedock and colleagues[27] observed that ~42% of hospitalized patients with COVID-19 were malnourished and the prevalence increased to ~67% in those admitted to ICU. It has been hypothesized that reduced food intake caused by COVID-19 symptoms (ie, anorexia, diarrhea, vomiting, nausea, abdominal pain, anosmia, and dysgeusia) and increased nutritional needs are main factors leading to malnutrition.[25,27,28] **Fig. 1** illustrates some of the mechanisms associated with muscle damage in individuals with long COVID.

CURRENT EVIDENCE

A summary of findings specifically related to body composition, muscle function, and QoL related to muscle health is shown in **Table 1**.

Muscle Mass and Other Body Composition Compartments

Body composition was assessed in 4 studies investigating long-term health sequelae of COVID-19 infection[29–32] using the following techniques: bioelectrical impedance analysis (BIA),[29,32] computed tomography (CT),[30] and ultrasound (US).[31]

After 4 to 5 weeks of COVID-19 infection, Tanriverdi and colleagues[32] assessed fat mass and fat-free mass (FFM) using BIA in people who recovered from mild (n = 25) and moderate (n = 23) disease severity. The 2 body compartments were not different between individuals who suffered mild or moderate disease, although a sex-specific comparison was not presented.[32] Another study assessed the body composition of patients discharged after COVID-19 using BIA.[29] Patients were classified according to disease severity (mild: n = 27; moderate: n = 51; severe: n = 26; critical: n = 20).[29] Fat-free mass index (FFMI) was calculated as $FFM/height^2$ and classified as low in 19% of the patients (7/27; 5/51; 7/26; 4/20).[29] No differences in FFMI or in the number of patients with low FFMI were observed among the 4 groups.[29]

In a prospective cohort study, 46 patients who were admitted to the ICU and received mechanical ventilation were assessed 3 months after hospital discharge.[30] Thoracic CT scans at the 12th vertebra were used to quantify skeletal muscle area, skeletal muscle radiation attenuation (an index of muscle quality), and intermuscular adipose tissue (IMAT).[30] Patients were categorized based on their performance on the 6-min walk distance (6MWD) test as having normal (n = 24) or low physical performance (<80% of predicted, n = 22).[30] Both skeletal muscle area and skeletal muscle radiation did not differ between patient subgroups; however, IMAT was higher in those with low physical performance.[30] Physical performance remained significantly

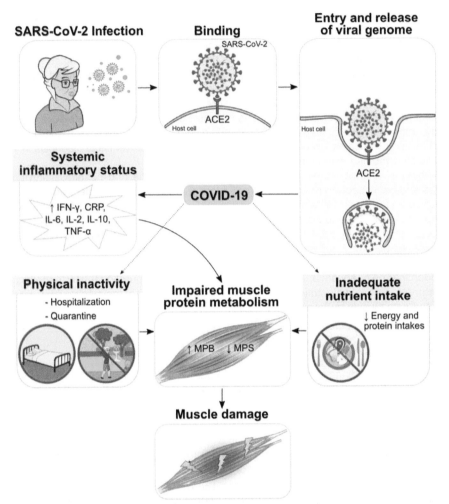

Fig. 1. Potential mechanisms of muscle damage in patients with long COVID-19. Systemic inflammatory state during the acute phase results in chronic release of proinflammatory cytokines, contributing to imbalances in muscle protein metabolism and impaired muscle health. In addition, physical inactivity due to hospitalization and quarantine as well as inadequate nutrition intake may also negatively impact muscle mass, quality, and function. (*From* Servier Medical Art. Servier. Available at https://smart.servier.com/; under Creative Commons Attribution 3.0 Unported License)

associated with IMAT after adjusting for age, sex, handgrip strength, and diffusing capacity for carbon monoxide.[30]

US images of the diaphragm muscle were assessed in 21 patients admitted to rehabilitation after severe COVID-19 and compared with 11 non–COVID-19 controls who needed ventilator support during hospitalization.[31] Diaphragm muscle thickness was not different between cases and controls, but the thickening ratio (ie, maximal inspiration/end-expiration) was reduced in patients who had been diagnosed with COVID-19, suggesting reduced diaphragm function.[31]

Table 1
Summary of findings related to body composition, muscle function, and quality of life related to muscle health in individuals with long COVID

Body Composition

Reference	Body Compartment	Technique	Timeline	Selected Main Findings
Tanriverdi et al,[32] 2021	FM and FFM	BIA	>3 mo after COVID-19	• No differences in FM and FFM by disease severity.
van den Borst et al,[29] 2021	FFMI	BIA	3 mo after COVID-19	• 19% had low FFMI, prevalence not different by disease severity.
van Gassel et al,[30] 2021	SMA, SMD, and IMAT	CT	3 mo after hospital discharge	• No differences in SMA and SMD between groups of physical performance. • IMAT was higher in patients with impaired physical performance.
Farr et al,[31] 2021	Diaphragm muscle thickness and thickening ratio	Ultrasound	Admitted to a rehabilitation after COVID-19	• Muscle thickness was not different between cases and controls. • Thickening ratio was reduced in patients with COVID-19.

Muscle Function

Reference	Muscle Function Evaluation	Assessment Test	Timeline	Selected Main Findings
van Gassel et al,[30] 2021	Muscle strength and physical performance	Handgrip strength	3 mo after COVID-19	• Trend for lower relative handgrip strength (no statistical difference in patients with impaired physical function).
Tanriverdi et al,[32] 2021	Muscle strength and physical performance	Handgrip and quadriceps muscle strength, and 4-m gait speed	>3 mo after COVID-19	• Disease severity did not relate to muscle weakness and function.
van den Borst et al,[29] 2021	Physical performance	6MWD	3 mo after COVID-19	• Greater impairment in individuals with moderate and severe disease.
Mittal et al,[33] 2021	Muscle strength	Handgrip strength	Not specified. Average: 3 mo	• Handgrip strength was significantly reduced in patients with COVID-19 with high fatigue scores.

(continued on next page)

Table 1
(continued)

Muscle Function			
Reference	**Muscle Function Evaluation**	**Assessment Test**	**Timeline**	**Selected Main Findings**

Reference	Muscle Function Evaluation	Assessment Test	Timeline	Selected Main Findings
Bellan et al,[34] 2021	Physical performance	SPPB and 2MWT	4- and 12-mo postdischarge	• 31.5% and 7.1% of patients had poor physical function at 4- and 12-mo follow-up. • Decrease in the prevalence of impaired physical performance at 12 mo.

Quality of Life			
Reference	**QOL Test**	**Timeline**	**Selected Main Findings**

Reference	QOL Test	Timeline	Selected Main Findings
van den Borst et al,[29] 2021	Nijmegen Clinical Screening Instrument	3 mo after COVID-19	• High prevalence of functional impairment, fatigue, and low QoL
van Gassel et al,[30] 2021	EQ-5D	3 mo after COVID-19	• Lower QoL in patients with impaired physical performance.
Cuerda et al,[35] 2021	EQ-5D-5 L	Ongoing study: patients are being followed for 12 mo	• 71.2% unable to move or with moderate impairment. • 75.5% with problems to perform daily activities.
Vaes et al,[36] 2021	EQ-5D-5 L	3 and 6 mo after COVID-19	• 62% with moderate-to-extreme problems performing daily activities.

Abbreviations: 6MWD, 6-minute walking distance; 2MWT, 2-minute walk test; BIA, bioelectrical impedance analysis; COVID-19, coronavirus disease, 2019; CT, computerized tomography; EQ-5D, European Quality of Life Five Dimension; EQ-5D-5L, 5-level European Quality of Life Five Dimension; FFMI, fat-free mass index; FFM, fat-free mass; FM, fat mass; IMAT, intermuscular adipose tissue; QoL, quality of life; SMA, skeletal muscle area; SMD, skeletal muscle radiodensity; SPPB, short physical performance battery.

Muscle Function

Muscle strength

Muscle strength was evaluated by handgrip strength testing in 3 studies assessing the health impact in individuals diagnosed with long COVID.[30,32,33] In a prospective cohort study, handgrip strength was assessed in 46 COVID-19 survivors 3 months after ICU discharge.[30] Individuals who tested lower than predicted on the 6MWD test showed a trend for lower handgrip strength than those with a normal 6MWD test result.[30]

Mittal and colleagues[33] compared handgrip strength of 52 patients with type 2 diabetes (T2D) who had mild to moderate COVID-19 and T2D patients who did not have COVID-19 (n = 56). Although no difference in strength was found between groups, handgrip strength was significantly reduced when patients with COVID-19 were categorized into high and low fatigue scores.[33] These findings indicate that neither patient group had significant dynapenia, but patients with T2D who had COVID-19 had higher fatigue and lower muscle strength than those who did not have COVID-19.

Handgrip strength and quadriceps muscle strength were assessed in a cross-sectional study including patients recovering from mild (n = 25) and moderate (n = 23) interstitial pneumonia after at least 12 weeks from COVID-19 diagnosis.[32] The prevalence of quadriceps and handgrip weakness was not different between groups (mild: 35%; moderate: 43.5%; P = .597).[32]

Physical performance

The prevalence of impaired physical performance in long COVID was evaluated in 4 studies including participants with different degrees of disease severity.[29,30,32,34] Direct measures of physical performance included walking tests (ie, 6MWD, 4-m gait speed test, and 2-min walk test)[29,30,32] and the short physical performance battery (SPPB).[34]

In a prospective observational study of mild to critical COVID-19 cases (n = 124), 22% of patients presented with low performance on the 6MWD test (ie, <80% of predicted) at 10 weeks after hospital discharge.[29] Although the prevalence of low 6MWD performance was numerically greater in individuals with moderate (28%) and severe (32%) compared with mild (12%) and critical (5%) disease, no statistical difference was found among groups, possibly due to the small sample size.[29] Using the same criteria to define impaired physical performance, another study observed that 48% of patients who survived critical COVID-19 had low performance on the 6MWD test at 3 months after hospital discharge.[30] Notably, the greater proportion of functional impairment observed in the latter study was likely driven by patients who required mechanical ventilation during ICU stay. Tanrivedi and colleagues[32] compared physical performance between groups of disease severity, and found that survivors of mild (n = 25) and moderate (n = 23) COVID-19 had similar 4-m gait speed.

The longest study evaluating physical performance in long COVID assessed 238 and 198 individuals after 4 and 12 months postdischarge, respectively.[34] Using a cutoff of 10 on the SPPB, low physical performance was found in 22.3% and 18.7% of patients at 4 and 12 months of follow-up, respectively. Highly functioning individuals (ie, those who scored 10 or more on the SPPB) also performed a 2-min walk test at both time points; 31.5% and 7.1% of patients had a poor physical function at 4 months and 12 months follow-up, respectively. Furthermore, the proportion of patients with low performance on either the SPPB or the 2-min walk test) was smaller at 12 months (25.8%) than at 4 months (52.8%).[34] This finding suggests that although some patients improved their physical function as they recovered, a significant proportion of individuals was still experiencing detrimental effects of COVID-19 after 12 months of hospital discharge.

Quality of Life Related to Muscle Health

QoL is related to several factors, and not only muscle health or physical performance. However, in this article, we focused only on studies assessing QoL related to muscle health. QoL of patients diagnosed with long COVID has been reported in 4 studies that assessed muscle function.[29,30,35,36] Two studies used the Euro-QoL-5D (EQ-5D) questionnaire.[30,36] This instrument evaluates 5 dimensions of a person's QoL (ie, mobility, self-care, daily activities, pain, and anxiety/depression).[30,35] Van Gassel and colleagues[30] assessed the QoL of 46 patients 3 months after hospital discharge using the EQ-5D. Health-related QoL was lower in people with low performance on the 6MWD test (n = 22) compared with those presenting with a normal test result (n = 24). The second study is an ongoing multicenter observational study including 176 COVID-19 survivors.[35] Preliminary results showed that 71.2% of participants were unable to move or presented with moderate impairment and 75.5% reported problems to perform daily activities.[35]

QoL of 239 patients with long COVID was assessed 3 and 6 months after the onset of COVID-19-related symptoms using the 5-level EuroQol-5 Dimensions version (EQ-5D-5 L).[36] This questionnaire is similar to the EQ-5D but with higher sensitivity[36]; 61.9% of the patients reported they were receiving physiotherapy and 11.7% rehabilitation between 3 and 6 months of follow-up. However, 62% of the patients still presented with moderate-to-extreme problems performing daily activities, and 49% experienced moderate-to-severe pain/discomfort.[36]

Lastly, QoL was assessed using the Nijmegen Clinical Screening Instrument in 124 patients with symptoms persisting for more than 6 weeks who attended a COVID-19 aftercare facility.[29] Patients were divided into 4 groups (mild: n = 27; moderate: n = 51; severe: n = 26; and critical: n = 20). Functional impairment was observed in 64% of the patients, fatigue in 69%, and reduced QoL in 72%.[29]

DISCUSSION

Long COVID has recently only been recognized; therefore, available evidence on the impact of this condition on muscle health is limited. Overall, studies suggest that long COVID negatively impacts body composition, muscle function, and QoL.

Body composition in individuals with long COVID was not found to differ based on disease severity.[29,30,32] However, this finding may be attributed to limitations of the body composition techniques used and small sample size, among others. Furthermore, the lack of body composition assessments during the acute phase and at hospital discharge hinders our understanding of whether people did experience changes in body composition, and at which disease phase. In one study, IMAT was found to be greater in patients with low physical performance.[30] This measurement is an estimate of skeletal muscle "quality" and has been associated with COVID-19 severity[37] and physical function after recovery.[38] Notably, long COVID was associated with a reduction of the thickening ratio of the diaphragm muscle, which can be related to diaphragm dysfunction.[31] This is an interesting marker in COVID-19 survivors, as it relates to fatigue after the acute phase.[39] In fact, 4 ongoing clinical trials are investigating how abnormal diaphragm muscle thickening ratio, which is related to muscle contractility, can impact QoL of individuals with long COVID.[40–43]

Muscle function of people with long COVID was shown to improve over 12 months.[34] The negative effects of long COVID on muscle function were obvious after 4 months and 12 months posthospital discharge,[32,34] although one study showed improvements at 1-year follow-up.[34] Inconsistency between the studies might be related to the degree of disease severity, age, and the presence of comorbidities.[44,45] Similarly to the findings observed by Huan and colleagues,[9] some studies hereby included reported worse physical performance in patients who recovered from severe COVID-19, when compared with those who had suffered a mild or moderate disease.[30,32,33] Notably, the presence of comorbidities also plays a critical role in long COVID. Cox and colleagues[46] observed that critically ill patients with low muscle mass who were recovering from sepsis experienced worse physical function 6 months after hospital discharge, when compared with critically ill patients with normal muscle mass. The presence of other comorbidities, such as obesity and pulmonary disease, has also been associated with symptoms of long COVID, including poor muscle function,[47] and is therefore an important variable to assess in future studies investigating long COVID.

Long COVID negatively affects QoL,[29,30,35,36] especially in individuals with impaired physical performance.[30] Some individuals still reported fatigue and difficulties in performing daily activities 6 months after hospital discharge and rehabilitation.[29,36] According to Rios and colleagues[48] and Rives-Lange,[49] malnutrition is a possible contributor to low QoL during long COVID. The relationship between QoL and nutritional status has been previously investigated in other conditions and is associated with impaired functional status and delayed recovery.[50] However, reduced QoL is not entirely explained by reduced physical performance, QoL also depends on mental and cognitive factors.[51]

Although older adults are at greater risk for the detrimental effects of long COVID on muscle health, little is known regarding age-related differences, and whether the sequelae are worse in older compared with younger adults. Age differences should be explored in future studies to better understand how long COVID affects muscle health across the lifespan.

Finally, despite the limited literature, long COVID directly or indirectly impacts muscle health. Muscle mass and function assessments can contribute toward the identification, diagnosis, and management of poor muscle health resulting from long COVID, consequently informing the design of targeted interventions.[52] Early approaches to optimize muscle health throughout disease trajectory and the recovery period are essential and should involve a multidisciplinary team of health professionals.

SUMMARY

Despite the relatively low number of studies and the presence of methodological limitations, available evidence suggests long COVID negatively impacts muscle health and QoL. These sequelae may be amplified in older adults due to preexisting age-related declines in muscle health. Acute and long-term assessments of these parameters are needed to optimize patient care. The mechanisms by which long COVID impacts muscle health are multifactorial and involve a combination of systemic inflammation, physical inactivity, poor nutritional status, and inadequate dietary intake. Other factors such as age, comorbidities, and degree of disease severity may also contribute to negative musculoskeletal outcomes during long COVID.

Overall, the evidence to date suggests long COVID negatively impacts body composition, muscle function, and QoL. Recovery and rehabilitation services with adequate nutrition, mental and social support should be explored as potential multimodal interventions to improve muscle health of these patients.

CLINICS CARE POINTS

- Clinicians should be aware of the prevalence and deleterious impact of poor muscle health in individuals with long COVID.

- People with long COVID can present with skeletal muscle symptoms 1 year after diagnosis.
- Muscle health in long COVID is related to low quality of life

DISCLOSURE

The authors have nothing to disclose.

REFERENCES

1. World Health Organization. (2021). A clinical case definition of post COVID-19 condition by a Delphi consensus, 6 October 2021. World Health Organization. Available at: https://apps.who.int/iris/handle/10665/345824. License: CC BY-NC-SA 3.0 IGO. Accessed January 28, 2022.
2. Greenhalgh T, Knight M, A'Court C, et al. Management of post-acute covid-19 in primary care. BMJ 2020;370:m3026.
3. NICE. Covid-19 rapid guideline: managing the long-term effects of covid-19. Available at: https://www.nice.org.uk/guidance/NG188. Accessed January 28, 2022.
4. Lopez-Leon S, Wegman-Ostrosky T, Perelman C, et al. More than 50 long-term effects of COVID-19: a systematic review and meta-analysis. Sci Rep 2021; 11(1):16144.
5. Soraas A, Kalleberg KT, Dahl JA, et al. Persisting symptoms three to eight months after non-hospitalized COVID-19, a prospective cohort study. PLoS One 2021; 16(8):e0256142.
6. Piotrowicz K, Gasowski J, Michel JP, et al. Post-COVID-19 acute sarcopenia: physiopathology and management. Aging Clin Exp Res 2021;33(10):2887–98.
7. Tieland M, Trouwborst I, Clark BC. Skeletal muscle performance and ageing. J Cachexia Sarcopenia Muscle 2018;9(1):3–19.
8. Karaarslan F, Guneri FD, Kardes S. Long COVID: rheumatologic/musculoskeletal symptoms in hospitalized COVID-19 survivors at 3 and 6 months. Clin Rheumatol 2022;41(1):289–96.
9. Huang C, Huang L, Wang Y, et al. 6-month consequences of COVID-19 in patients discharged from hospital: a cohort study. Lancet 2021;397(10270): 220–32.
10. Akbarialiabad H, Taghrir MH, Abdollahi A, et al. Long COVID, a comprehensive systematic scoping review. Infection 2021;49(6):1163–86.
11. Docherty AB, Harrison EM, Green CA, et al. Features of 20 133 UK patients in hospital with covid-19 using the ISARIC WHO Clinical Characterisation Protocol: prospective observational cohort study. BMJ 2020;369:m1985.
12. Welch C, Greig C, Masud T, et al. COVID-19 and acute sarcopenia. Aging Dis 2020;11(6):1345–51.
13. Benton DJ, Wrobel AG, Xu P, et al. Receptor binding and priming of the spike protein of SARS-CoV-2 for membrane fusion. Nature 2020;588(7837): 327–30.
14. Hoffmann M, Kleine-Weber H, Schroeder S, et al. SARS-CoV-2 cell entry depends on ACE2 and TMPRSS2 and is blocked by a clinically proven protease Inhibitor. Cell 2020;181(2):271–80.e8.
15. Disser NP, De Micheli AJ, Schonk MM, et al. Musculoskeletal consequences of COVID-19. J Bone Joint Surg Am 2020;102(14):1197–204.
16. Finsterer J, Scorza FA. SARS-CoV-2 myopathy. J Med Virol 2021;93(4):1852–3.

17. Malik P, Patel K, Pinto C, et al. Post-acute COVID-19 syndrome (PCS) and health-related quality of life (HRQoL)-A systematic review and meta-analysis. J Med Virol 2022;94(1):253–62.
18. Liu J, Li S, Liu J, et al. Longitudinal characteristics of lymphocyte responses and cytokine profiles in the peripheral blood of SARS-CoV-2 infected patients. EBio-Medicine 2020;55:102763.
19. Webster JM, Kempen LJAP, Hardy RS, et al. Inflammation and skeletal muscle wasting during cachexia. Front Physiol 2020;11:597675.
20. Pretorius E, Vlok M, Venter C, et al. Persistent clotting protein pathology in Long COVID/Post-Acute Sequelae of COVID-19 (PASC) is accompanied by increased levels of antiplasmin. Cardiovasc Diabetol 2021;20(1):172.
21. Theobald SJ, Simonis A, Georgomanolis T, et al. Long-lived macrophage reprog-ramming drives spike protein-mediated inflammasome activation in COVID-19. EMBO Mol Med 2021;13(8):e14150.
22. Schefold JC, Wollersheim T, Grunow JJ, et al. Muscular weakness and muscle wasting in the critically ill. J Cachexia Sarcopenia Muscle 2020;11(6):1399–412.
23. Soares MN, Eggelbusch M, Naddaf E, et al. Skeletal muscle alterations in pa-tients with acute Covid-19 and post-acute sequelae of Covid-19. J Cachexia Sar-copenia Muscle 2022;13(1):11–22.
24. Doykov I, Hällqvist J, Gilmour KC, et al. The long tail of Covid-19' - the detection of a prolonged inflammatory response after a SARS-CoV-2 infection in asymptom-atic and mildly affected patients. F1000Res 2020;9:1349.
25. Barazzoni R, Bischoff SC, Breda J, et al. ESPEN expert statements and practical guidance for nutritional management of individuals with SARS-CoV-2 infection. Clin Nutr (Edinburgh, Scotland) 2020;39(6):1631–8.
26. Gerard M, Mahmutovic M, Malgras A, et al. Long-term Evolution of malnutrition and loss of muscle strength after COVID-19: a major and Neglected Component of long COVID-19. Nutrients 2021;13(11):3964.
27. Bedock D, Bel Lassen P, Mathian A, et al. Prevalence and severity of malnutrition in hospitalized COVID-19 patients. Clin Nutr ESPEN 2020;40:214–9.
28. Wischmeyer PE. Nutrition therapy in sepsis. Crit Care Clin 2018;34(1):107–25.
29. van den Borst B, Peters JB, Brink M, et al. Comprehensive health assessment 3 Months after recovery from acute Coronavirus disease 2019 (COVID-19). Clin Infect Dis 2021;73(5):e1089–98.
30. van Gassel RJJ, Bels J, Remij L, et al. Functional outcomes and their association with physical performance in mechanically ventilated Coronavirus disease 2019 survivors at 3 Months following hospital discharge: a cohort study. Crit Care Med 2021;49(10):1726–38.
31. Farr E, Wolfe AR, Deshmukh S, et al. Diaphragm dysfunction in severe COVID-19 as determined by neuromuscular ultrasound. Ann Clin Transl Neurol 2021;8(8):1745–9.
32. Tanriverdi A, Savci S, Kahraman BO, et al. Extrapulmonary features of post-COVID-19 patients: muscle function, physical activity, mood, and sleep quality. Ir J Med Sci 2021;1–7. https://doi.org/10.1007/s11845-021-02667-3.
33. Mittal J, Ghosh A, Bhatt SP, et al. High prevalence of post COVID-19 fatigue in patients with type 2 diabetes: a case-control study. Diabetes Metab Syndr 2021;15(6):102302.
34. Bellan M, Soddu D, Balbo PE, et al. Respiratory and psychophysical sequelae among patients with COVID-19 four months after hospital discharge. JAMA Netw Open 2021;4(1):e2036142.

35. Cuerda C, Sanchez Lopez I, Gil Martinez C, et al. Impact of COVID-19 in nutritional and functional status of survivors admitted in intensive care units during the first outbreak. Preliminary results of the NUTRICOVID study. Clin Nutr 2021. https://doi.org/10.1016/j.clnu.2021.11.017. S0261-5614(21)00526-4.
36. Vaes AW, Goertz YMJ, Van Herck M, et al. Recovery from COVID-19: a sprint or marathon? 6-month follow-up data from online long COVID-19 support group members. ERJ Open Res 2021;7(2). 00141-2021.
37. Viddeleer AR, Raaphorst J, Min M, et al. Intramuscular adipose tissue at level Th12 is associated with survival in COVID-19. J Cachexia Sarcopenia Muscle 2021;12(3):823–7.
38. Besutti G, Pellegrini M, Ottone M, et al. The impact of chest CT body composition parameters on clinical outcomes in COVID-19 patients. PLOS ONE 2021;16(5): e0251768.
39. Shi Z, de Vries HJ, Vlaar APJ, et al. Diaphragm pathology in critically ill patients with COVID-19 and postmortem findings from 3 medical Centers. JAMA Intern Med 2021;181(1):122–4.
40. ClinicalTrials.gov. National Library of Medicine (U.S.). Respiratory Muscles After Hospitalisation for COVID-19 (REMAP-COVID-19) .Identifier NCT04854863. Available from: https://clinicaltrials.gov/ct2/show/NCT04854863?cond= NCT04854863&draw=2&rank=1
41. ClinicalTrials.gov. National Library of Medicine (U.S.). Diaphragm Ultrasound Evaluation During Weaning From Mechanical Ventilation in the Positive COVID-19 Patient. Identifier NCT05019313. Available from:https://clinicaltrials.gov/ct2/show/NCT05019313?cond=NCT05019313&draw=2&rank=1
42. ClinicalTrials.gov. National Library of Medicine (U.S.).Pulmonary Function in Patients Recovering From COVID19 Infection : a Pilot Study (EFRUPIC). Identifier NCT05074927. Available from: https://clinicaltrials.gov/ct2/show/NCT05074927? cond=NCT05074927&draw=2&rank=1
43. ClinicalTrials.gov. National Library of Medicine (U.S.). Respiratory Muscle Function, Dyspnea, Exercise Capacity and Quality of Life in Severe COVID19 Patients. Identifier NCT04853940. Available from: https://clinicaltrials.gov/ct2/show/ NCT04853940?cond=NCT04853940&draw=2&rank=1
44. Kirwan R, McCullough D, Butler T, et al. Sarcopenia during COVID-19 lockdown restrictions: long-term health effects of short-term muscle loss. GeroScience 2020;42(6):1547–78.
45. Liu Y, Mao B, Liang S, et al. Association between age and clinical characteristics and outcomes of COVID-19. Eur Respir J 2020;55(5):2001112.
46. Cox MC, Booth M, Ghita G, et al. The impact of sarcopenia and acute muscle mass loss on long-term outcomes in critically ill patients with intra-abdominal sepsis. J Cachexia Sarcopenia Muscle 2021;12(5):1203–13.
47. Aminian A, Bena J, Pantalone KM, et al. Association of obesity with postacute sequelae of COVID-19. Diabetes Obes Metab 2021;23(9):2183–8.
48. Rios TC, de Oliveira LPM, da Costa MLV, et al. A poorer nutritional status impacts quality of life in a sample population of elderly cancer patients. Health Qual Life Outcomes 2021;19(1):90.
49. Rives-Lange C, Zimmer A, Merazka A, et al. Evolution of the nutritional status of COVID-19 critically-ill patients: a prospective observational study from ICU admission to three months after ICU discharge. Clin Nutr 2021. https://doi.org/ 10.1016/j.clnu.2021.05.007. S0261-5614(21)00257-0.
50. Norman K, Kirchner H, Lochs H, et al. Malnutrition affects quality of life in gastroenterology patients. World J Gastroenterol 2006;12(21):3380–5.

51. Geense WW, de Graaf M, Vermeulen H, et al. Reduced quality of life in ICU survivors - the story behind the numbers: a mixed methods study. J Crit Care 2021; 65:36–41.
52. Prado CM, Anker SD, Coats AJS, et al. Nutrition in the spotlight in cachexia, sarcopenia and muscle: avoiding the wildfire. J Cachexia Sarcopenia Muscle 2021; 12(1):3–8.

Malnutrition and Sarcopenia in COVID-19 Survivors

Stefan Grund, MD[a,b], Jürgen M. Bauer, MD, PhD[a,b],*

KEYWORDS

- Sarcopenia • Malnutrition • COVID-19 survivors • Long COVID • Nursing home

KEY POINTS

- Malnutrition and sarcopenia are both highly prevalent among older COVID-19 survivors.
- Admission to intensive care in older hospital patients and delirium in nursing home residents are negative predictors for both syndromes.
- Routine monitoring of nutritional and functional status is indicated in all older COVID-19 survivors.
- Individually adapted geriatric rehabilitation should be provided especially for those that are at risk for loss of independence.

The observation that nutritional status and functionality are deeply intertwined in older persons holds especially true in the context of the COVID-19 pandemic. One of the key symptoms of infections with the SARS-CoV-2 virus has been its negative impact on taste and smell thereby significantly decreasing the attractiveness of adequate food intake in infected older individuals.[1] As this sensory deficit may persist for several months the nutritional status of older patients with post–COVID-19 may be severely impaired. In acute hospital patients, the risk of malnutrition has been linked to the severity of the infection, while in the subacute and chronic stage of the disease inadequate food intake may also be seen in patients that are not affected by a serious course of the disease. Inadequate intake of calories and protein has been established as one of the main etiologic factors of sarcopenia, that in patients with COVID-19 often combines with the deleterious effects of immobilization and inflammation. For these reasons, functional status and overall prognosis may be negatively affected in older COVID-19 survivors. With this article, we will provide some additional insight into the specifics of this patient population.

a Center for Geriatric Medicine, Heidelberg University, Rohrbacher Strasse 149, 69126 Heidelberg, Germany; b Agaplesion Bethanien Hospital, Rohrbacher Strasse 149, 69126 Heidelberg, Germany
* Corresponding author. Rohrbacher Str. 149, Heidelberg 69126, Germany.
E-mail address: juergen.bauer@agaplesion.de

Clin Geriatr Med 38 (2022) 559–564
https://doi.org/10.1016/j.cger.2022.04.001
0749-0690/22/© 2022 Elsevier Inc. All rights reserved.

MALNUTRITION IN DIFFERENT HEALTH CARE SETTINGS
Hospital and Ambulatory Setting During Acute Disease

During the acute stage of the disease each of 407 Dutch patients with COVID-19 hospital (mean age 64y) had at least one nutritional complaint (**Box 1**).[2] Among those were decreased appetite in 58% and the feeling of being full in 49%. One in 3 patients experienced a change in taste, loss of taste, and/or loss of smell. In this study, 35% of the patients were diagnosed as being malnourished.

With regard to the subacute stage of the disease, it was shown in a French study that 30 days after hospital discharge (D30) 33.3% of respondents (mean age 60 years) were malnourished with 13.2% fulfilling the criteria of severe malnutrition and 20.1% fulfilling those of moderate malnutrition[3,4]. In this study, severe malnutrition was defined as weight loss > 10% compared to the weight before COVID-19 or a BMI less than 17 kg/m^2 (<18.5 for patients >70 year old). Moderate malnutrition was defined as weight loss > 5% compared to the weight before COVID-19 or BMI less than 18.5 kg/m2 (<21 for patients >70 year old). 23.2% had been malnourished at discharge, but were no longer malnourished at D30. A higher risk for persistent malnutrition was associated with admission to ICU, subjective functional loss at discharge, and male sex. In this study, it was also shown that subjective functional loss was present in 76.8% of patients at discharge and in 26.2% still at D30.

Additional follow-up data for the above patient population were published by Gérard and colleagues.[5] Six months after discharge 36% (43/119) of respondents fulfilled the criteria for persistent malnutrition, 14.3% (17/119) described persistent subjective functional loss, and 14.9% (18/119) a reduced performance status. Obesity and admission to intensive care were both identified as risk factors for persistent functional impairments.

In the above-cited study by Wierdsma and colleagues, appetite reduction was still evident in 30% of patients 3 to 5 months after discharge. In this population, severity of illness and admission to intensive care were associated with the persistence of complaints.[2]

Box 1
Nutrition-related complaints among hospital patients with COVID-19

Decreased appetite and loss of appetite

Feeling of being full

Change in taste

Loss of taste

Loss of smell

Tiredness (assistance with eating required)

Swallowing difficulties and/or dysphagia

Nausea

Vomiting

Chewing difficulties

Pain in the oral cavity

Adapted from Wierdsma NJ, Kruizenga HM, Konings LA, et al. Poor nutritional status, risk of sarcopenia and nutrition related complaints are prevalent in COVID-19 patients during and after hospital admission. Clin Nutr ESPEN. 2021;43:369–376. https://doi.org/10.1016/j.clnesp.2021.03.021; with permission

Taking into account the persistent nature of malnutrition in patients with COVID-19 that were admitted to hospital during the acute course of disease, it will be indicated to routinely assess their nutritional status before discharge and to monitor it regularly during the first post–COVID-19 year. Nutritional interventions should be started early after diagnosis of malnutrition and preventive measures should be initiated in those that are at high risk for developing it during the course of the disease, especially in those patients that are admitted to intensive care. There have been first indications that this approach may allow for good results in younger patient populations.[6] At the moment it remains to be proven to what extent these positive results can be reproduced in older multimorbid patients with COVID-19.

The Nursing Home Setting

In a US study that focused on nursing home residents, it was shown that early during an outbreak of COVID-19 17.9% showed symptoms of anorexia and that this percentage increased to 70.8% after 21 days.[7] This increase of anorexia symptoms was paralleled by a significant increase of delirium in patients with COVID-19, which increased from 18.6% to 56% during the same period. Therefore, it may be reasoned that the presence of delirium aggravated anorectic symptoms in this patient population. However, it should also be considered that insufficient nutritional intake may have triggered delirium. This two-way relationship has already been addressed in two recent articles.[8,9] Considering the above the presence of delirium warrants special consideration in the context of malnutrition in older nursing home patients with COVID-19.

Focusing on the subacute course of COVID-19 in older nursing home residents, Martinchek et all demonstrated that there was a mean weight loss of 4.6% (3.5 kg) in patients with COVID-19 2 months after the onset of COVID-19-related symptoms.[10]

It also seems important to mention that preventive restrictions during a local outbreak[10] and general contact restrictions for nursing homes during the pandemic[11] can have a negative impact on the nutritional status including weight loss of COVID-19 negative residents. However, the respective consequences seem to be less severe than in those that have been infected by the coronavirus.[10] In this context psychological factors and a lack of mealtime assistance may be of special relevance.

Summarizing the above, nursing home residents are in general at a high risk of deteriorating nutritional status during the pandemic. Food and fluid intake deserves special attention in positive residents with signs of delirium.

SARCOPENIA

From a subacute and chronic perspective, an inadequate intake of calories and protein will lead to a decrease in muscle mass and subsequently to a loss of strength and function. This process may finally cause overt sarcopenia in patients with post–COVID-19. However, in those that have been affected by a more serious course of disease, sarcopenia may be present already before hospital discharge. Systemic inflammation, immobilization, hypoxemia, and malnutrition may all cause loss of muscle mass and function, while the relative contribution of the etiologic factors may vary to the relevant degree.[12] In this context it also has to be appreciated that the presence of sarcopenia in patients with COVID-19 already early after admission to hospital has been identified as an independent prognostic parameter that was associated with length of stay.[13]

A study from Spain which was based on data from the first COVID-19 wave focused on the nutritional and functional status of COVID-19 survivors, average age of 60 years, who had been treated in intensive care units.[14] The study participants had suffered an average weight loss of 16.6% during their hospital stay. While 83.5% were at risk of malnutrition at discharge, 86.9% were at risk of sarcopenia based on the SARC-F questionnaire. Those latter groups had a longer length of hospital and ICU stay than those patients that were not at risk. Furthermore, they had received tracheostomy and invasive ventilation more often. 86.3% of those at risk of sarcopenia showed moderate or total dependency according to the Barthel-Index at discharge, while the respective percentage was only 34.8% in those that were not at risk. Although nutritional therapy would have been warranted in a high percentage of those patients it was prescribed only in 38%, mainly in form of oral nutritional supplements.

The high probability of being at risk of sarcopenia among hospital patients admitted with COVID-19 has been confirmed in a recent study from the Netherlands, that also included non-ICU patients. In this study, the SARC-F indicated a risk of sarcopenia in 73% of all included patients (mean age of 64.8 years).[2]

Reflecting on the presented data some critical comments seem to be justified. In both trials, the SARC-F was applied to hospital patients during the acute course of disease before discharge. Under these circumstances, there might have been a relevant overlap with conditions that affect functionality but that are not closely related to sarcopenia, like partial respiratory insufficiency or acute and subacute cognitive impairment. In addition, the above studies do not provide an estimate of muscle mass in their patient populations. The follow-up of the study by Wierdsma showed that the percentage of patients at risk of sarcopenia fell from 72% at discharge to 21% between 4 and 7 weeks after discharge. This decrease in prevalence would not be expected in truly sarcopenic patients. Correctly the authors only referred to a risk of sarcopenia and not to the diagnosis of sarcopenia. However, it is absolutely obvious that COVID-19 infections in older hospital patients may trigger the development of sarcopenia or worsen already existing sarcopenia, primarily as a consequence of immobilization, malnutrition, and inflammation. Unfortunately, we may not have sufficient information to calculate the precise prevalence of sarcopenia in older COVID-19 survivors at this moment. Therefore, it may be more adequate to describe the decline of functionality and resulting dependence in activities of daily living in this population without applying the diagnosis of sarcopenia.

In an Italian study reporting on 34 patients with post–acute COVID-19, mean age 70 years, that were admitted to rehabilitation 20 patients (58%) were diagnosed as being sarcopenic based on the EWGSOP criteria.[15] When compared with the nonsarcopenic patients they showed slightly higher age (71.5 vs 68 years), lower BMI values (21 vs 27.3. kg/m^2) and significantly higher ferritin and lower vitamin D values.

Additional factors may contribute to the development of sarcopenia in the subacute and chronic course of the disease. While it is still unclear whether viral infiltration of the muscle affects its function directly, for example, by the impairment of its mitochondria,

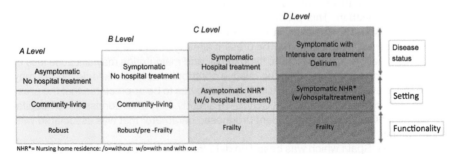

NHR*= Nursing home residence: /o=without: w/o=with and with out

Fig. 1. Level of risk for the persistence of malnutrition and sarcopenia in older COVID-19 survivors–A proposed model.

indirect mechanisms have been shown to be of relevance. In this context, the contribution of prolonged disuse should be regarded as a key factor. The postviral chronic fatigue syndrome may be diagnosed in a relevant percentage of patients with COVID-19. It has been characterized by profound fatigue, sleep disturbances, neurocognitive changes, and postexertional malaise. In a recent systematic review fatigue was present in 32% of patients with COVID-19 12 weeks and beyond after diagnosis of the infection.[16] In addition, the proportion of individuals exhibiting cognitive impairment was 22% in the same analysis. Fatigue and cognitive impairment may both significantly contribute to the disuse of the muscle in patients with post–COVID-19.

SUMMARY

Malnutrition has been one of the most common complications of older COVID-19 survivors. COVID-19 associated symptoms like loss of appetite as well as changes in taste and smell may trigger the deterioration of nutritional status, while other complications of the disease may contribute to it, like respiratory failure that necessitates admission to the ICU. Especially in nursing home residents reduced food intake may be related to preexisting and also to incident geriatric syndromes like delirium. Sarcopenia has also been highly prevalent in older COVID-19 survivors. It is caused and exacerbated by COVID-19-associated inflammatory processes, total or partial immobilization, and malnutrition. COVID-19 survivors may be at high risk of developing the vicious circle that results from the interaction of deteriorating nutritional status and declining functionality. A model for general risk assessment in older COVID-19 survivors with regard to the persistence of malnutrition and sarcopenia is proposed in **Fig. 1**. Regular monitoring of nutritional and functional status isindicated in all older COVID-19 survivors. When malnutrition and/or functional decline have been identified in this patient population, low-threshold provision of individualized nutritional and exercise interventions should be installed. In those that are most seriously affected by malnutrition and sarcopenia ambulatory or inpatient rehabilitation has to be considered. Geriatric rehabilitation programs should be specifically adapted to the needs of older patients with COVID-19.

CLINICS CARE POINTS

- All older COVID-19 survivors should be screened repeatedly for malnutrition and sarcopenia after the acute disease.
- Delirium in COVID-19 survivors warrants special awareness in this regard.
- Nutritional intervention should be started early during the disease, if indicated.
- The repeated assessment of functionality should trigger the allocation of rehabilitative care in older COVID-19 survivors.

REFERENCES

1. Agyeman AA, Chin KL, Landersdorfer CB, et al. Smell and taste dysfunction in patients with COVID-19: a systematic review and meta-analysis. Mayo Clin Proc 2020;95:1621–31.
2. Wierdsma NJ, Kruizenga HM, Konings LA, et al. Poor nutritional status, risk of sarcopenia and nutrition related complaints are prevalent in COVID-19 patients during and after hospital admission. Clin Nutr ESPEN 2021;43:369–76.

3. Quilliot D, Gérard M, Bonsack O, et al. Impact of severe SARS-CoV-2 infection on nutritional status and subjective functional loss in a prospective cohort of COVID-19 survivors. BMJ Open 2021;11(7):e048948.

4. Saniasiaya J, Islam MA, Abdullah B. Prevalence of olfactory dysfunction in coronavirus disease 2019 (COVID-19): a meta-analysis of 27,492 patients. Laryngoscope 2021;131(4):865–78.

5. Gérard M, Mahmutovic M, Malgras A, et al. Long-term evolution of malnutrition and loss of muscle strength after COVID-19: a major and neglected component of long COVID-19. Nutrients 2021;13(11):3964.

6. Bedock D, Couffignal J, Bel Lassen P, et al. Evolution of nutritional status after early nutritional management in COVID-19 hospitalized patients. Nutrients 2021;13(7):2276.

7. Shi SM, Bakaev I, Chen H, et al. Risk factors, presentation, and course of coronavirus disease 2019 in a large, academic long-term care facility. J Am Med Dir Assoc 2020;21(10):1378–83.

8. Morandi A, Pozzi C, Milisen K, et al. An interdisciplinary statement of scientific societies for the advancement of delirium care across Europe (EDA, EANS, EUGMS, COTEC, IPTOP/WCPT). BMC Geriatr 2019;19(1):253.

9. Mudge A, Young A, Cahill M, et al. Nutrition and delirium. In: Geirsdóttir ÓG, Bell JJ, editors. Interdisciplinary nutritional management and care for older adults. Perspectives in nursing management and care for older adults. Cham: Springer; 2021. https://doi.org/10.1007/978-3-030-63892-4_19.

10. Martinchek M, Beiting KJ, Walker J, et al. Weight loss in COVID-19-positive nursing home residents. J Am Med Dir Assoc 2021;22(2):257–8.

11. Danilovich MK, Norrick CR, Hill KC, et al. Nursing home resident weight loss during coronavirus disease 2019 restrictions. J Am Med Dir Assoc 2020;21(11):1568–9.

12. Soares MN, Eggelbusch M, Naddaf E, et al. Skeletal muscle alterations in patients with acute Covid-19 and post-acute sequelae of Covid-19. J Cachexia Sarcopenia Muscle 2022. https://doi.org/10.1002/jcsm.12896.

13. Kim JW, Yoon JS, Kim EJ, et al. Prognostic implication of baseline sarcopenia for length of hospital stay and survival in patients with coronavirus Disease 2019. J Gerontol A Biol Sci Med Sci 2021;76(8):e110–6.

14. Cuerda C, Sánchez López I, Gil Martinez C, et al. NUTRICOVID study research group of SENDIMAD. impact of COVID-19 in nutritional and functional status of survivors admitted in intensive care units during the first outbreak. Preliminary results of the NUTRICOVID study. Clin Nutr 2021. https://doi.org/10.1016/j.clnu.2021.11.017.

15. Gobbi M, Bezzoli E, Ismelli F, et al. Skeletal muscle mass, sarcopenia and rehabilitation outcomes in post-acute COVID-19 patients. J Clin Med 2021;10(23):5623.

16. Ceban F, Ling S, Lui LMW, et al. Fatigue and cognitive impairment in Post-COVID-19 Syndrome: a systematic review and meta-analysis. Brain Behav Immun 2022;101:93–135.

Nutraceuticals and Dietary Supplements for Older Adults with Long COVID-19

Matteo Tosato, MD, PhD[a], Francesca Ciciarello, MD[a],
Maria Beatrice Zazzara, MD[a], Cristina Pais, MD[a],
Giulia Savera, MSc[a], Anna Picca, PhD[a], Vincenzo Galluzzo, MD[a],
Hélio José Coelho-Júnior, PhD[b], Riccardo Calvani, PhD[a,*],
Emanuele Marzetti, MD, PhD[a,b], Francesco Landi, MD, PhD[a,b], on
behalf of Gemelli Against COVID-19 Post-Acute Care Team

KEYWORDS

- Geriatrics • Gerontology • Frailty • Sarcopenia • Fatigue • Nutrition
- Bioactive foods • Therapy

KEY POINTS

- Long-term persistence of COVID-19–related symptoms after SARS-CoV-2 infection impacts quality of life.
- Several mechanisms may be involved in the persistence of COVID-19 symptoms, including chronic inflammation, immunometabolic processes, endothelial dysfunction, and gut dysbiosis.
- Bioactive foods, supplements, and nutraceuticals may be used for the management of long-term COVID-19 clinical sequelae.

INTRODUCTION

SARS-CoV-2 infection affects multiple organs owing to the ubiquitous distribution of its target receptor ACE-2.[1] Increasing interest has been paid to the postacute phase of COVID-19. The time to recover from an acute COVID-19 episode ranges from 2 to 6 weeks depending on disease severity.[2] However, a substantial share of people reports clinical sequelae weeks or months after symptom onset. This condition, known as postacute COVID-19 syndrome, postacute sequelae of COVID-19, or long COVID syndrome, encompasses long-lasting signs and symptoms, such as cough, dyspnea,

[a] Fondazione Policlinico Universitario "Agostino Gemelli" IRCCS, L.go A. Gemelli 8, Rome 00168, Italy; [b] Department of Geriatrics and Orthopedics, Università Cattolica del Sacro Cuore, L.go F. Vito 8, Rome 00168, Italy
* Corresponding author.
E-mail address: riccardo.calvani@policlinicogemelli.it

Clin Geriatr Med 38 (2022) 565–591
https://doi.org/10.1016/j.cger.2022.04.004
0749-0690/22/© 2022 Elsevier Inc. All rights reserved.

fatigue, difficulties with memory and concentration ("brain fog"), sleep disorders, gastrointestinal complaints, and musculoskeletal problems.[3,4]

A recent systematic review showed that more than half of COVID-19 survivors (mostly middle-aged men hospitalized during the acute phase) had at least one long-lasting symptom at 6 months.[5] Results from a digital questionnaire in a cohort of middle-aged nonhospitalized patients with COVID-19 from Denmark showed that persistent symptoms lasting for more than 4 weeks were experienced by 36% of participants who had been symptomatic during the acute phase.[6] Recently, our group showed that persisting symptoms were common in older adults who had been hospitalized for COVID-19, with approximately 50% of the sample presenting with 3 or more symptoms after 3 months of hospital discharge.[7] Symptom persistence was more frequent in those who experienced fatigue during acute COVID-19.

The mechanisms of chronic COVID-19 manifestations have not been yet unveiled. Several hypotheses are currently being tested.[4,8] These include viral persistence associated with chronic inflammation, autoimmune processes, alterations in immunometabolic pathways, dysbiosis, endothelial damage, and unresolved organ damage.[3,4,8] It is noteworthy that some of the immunologic and systemic features of long COVID resemble signs of accelerated or premature aging, and may aggravate pre-existing age-associated degenerative conditions, such as sarcopenia and cognitive decline.[9-11]

Specific treatments for long COVID are currently lacking. Patient management mostly relies on symptomatic treatments and recommendations to conduct an active and healthy lifestyle. A plethora of dietary supplements and natural bioactive substances have been tested for their potential to contrast long COVID.[12,13] In this review, the possible actions of nutraceuticals and dietary supplements on mechanisms associated with long COVID are described. A brief overview of ongoing studies investigating the effects of specific nutraceuticals in patients with long COVID attending the outpatient service at the Fondazione Policlinico A. Gemelli IRCCS (Rome, Italy)[14] is presented.

DISCUSSION
Amino Acids

Amino acids play a crucial role in cell metabolism and modulate several biological processes (eg, inflammation, glucose homeostasis, redox balance) that may be involved in post-COVID clinical sequelae.[4,8,15] Amino acids support the increased metabolic demands of activated immune cells by contributing critical intermediates to biosynthetic and energy-producing pathways, such as glycolysis, tricarboxylic acid (TCA) cycle, and oxidative phosphorylation pathways.[15]

Glutamine replenishes TCA cycle intermediates that have been consumed in biosynthetic processes in T cells, macrophages, and plasma cells through anaplerosis.[16-18] In immune cells, glutamine is also used for glutathione and in hexosamine biosynthetic pathways and supplies amino groups for other amino acids via transamination.[19]

The branched-chain amino acids (BCAAs) leucine, isoleucine, and valine are essential amino acids with well-established effects on protein synthesis and glucose homeostasis. BCAAs mainly act through the stimulation of cellular anabolic signaling pathways (eg, phosphoinositide 3-kinase-protein kinase B, mammalian target of rapamycin [mTOR]).[20] BCAAs may exert direct and indirect effects on immune function.[15] In vitro models have shown that BCAAs are essential for proliferating lymphocytes to synthesize proteins and nucleotides in response to stimulation.[21] BCAAs can be incorporated into and oxidized by immune cells. The amount of BCAAs incorporated into proteins is higher in lymphocytes, followed by eosinophils and neutrophils.[21] In immune cells, BCAAs are also sources of the coenzyme A (CoA) derivatives acetyl-CoA and succinyl-CoA, which enter the TCA cycle and support mitochondrial bioenergetics.[15] BCAAs may also improve gut mucosal surface defense by stimulating soluble immunoglobulin A secretion.[22]

Arginine is a semiessential amino acid involved in multiple biological processes. Its main activities on the immune system derive from its conversion to nitric oxide (NO) by NO synthase (NOS) and its metabolism through arginase, that competes with NOS for arginine availability in most immune cells.[23] NO is known to have direct and indirect antiviral activity through the generation of immunomodulatory oxidized phospholipids.[24–26] NO also exerts potent anti-inflammatory effects via inhibition of leukocyte recruitment.[27,28] Several studies in animal models have shown that the mechanisms of NO action on leukocyte function involve the activation of guanylyl cyclase, followed by the generation of cyclic GMP that suppresses the expression of P-selectin, a crucial mediator in leukocyte adhesion.[29] Reduced arginine bioavailability may impair T-cell response and function.[30] In patients with COVID-19, a decrease in plasma arginine levels with concomitant increase in arginase activity was associated with impaired T-cell proliferative capacity, which can be restored in vitro by arginine supplementation.[31] Arginine, through its action on NO synthesis, may also modulate endothelial and respiratory functions and exert antithrombotic and cytoprotective activities.[32] Preliminary data suggest that oral arginine supplementation added to standard therapy reduced the need of respiratory support and the duration of in-hospital stay in patients with severe COVID-19.[33] Because of its modulating activities on inflammation and endothelial function, arginine has also been indicated as a plausible agent to contrast COVID-19 sequelae.

Collectively, available evidence suggests that amino acids are crucial to modulate immune response and several other mechanisms involved in both acute and chronic COVID-19. In older adults, the physiologic changes associated with the aging process (eg, increased splanchnic extraction, anabolic resistance, chronic inflammation) may further increase the need of adequate amino acid supplies.[34] Protein/amino acid malnutrition in older adults is associated with immune dysfunction and sarcopenia, the latter being aggravated by reduced mobility and inflammatory processes induced by COVID-19.[35]

Given these premises, it is reasonable to focus on the achievement of an adequate amino acid intake in COVID-19 survivors, also through oral supplementation. In particular, amino acid intake should be monitored in older people who are at greater risk of malnutrition as a specific consequence of SARS-CoV-2 infection.

Hydroxy-Beta-Methylbutyrate

Beta-hydroxy-beta-methyl butyrate (HMB) is the active metabolite of leucine.[36] HMB, through the stimulation of mTOR-dependent pathways, modulates several physiologic processes, including protein metabolism, insulin activity, skeletal muscle hypertrophy, cell apoptosis, and muscle stem cell proliferation and differentiation.[37]

Oral supplementation of HMB (3 g/d) mitigates the decline in muscle mass and preserves muscle function in older adults and frail people, especially during hospital stay and recovery.[38] Interestingly, HMB may modulate the immune and inflammatory response, especially under stressful conditions.[39] HMB supplementation was found to have short-term anti-inflammatory and anticatabolic effects and to improve pulmonary function in patients with chronic obstructive pulmonary disease in an intensive care unit setting.[40]

Possible effects of HMB on brain have also been explored, starting from the evidence that HMB crosses the blood-brain barrier in rats.[41] HMB was found to promote neurite outgrowth in vitro,[42] and long-term HMB supplementation in rats attenuated age-related dendritic shrinkage of pyramidal neurons in the medial prefrontal cortex,[43] thus suggesting possible beneficial effects on cognition.[44,45]

Based on its well-established effects on muscle mass preservation and its potential biological activities on physiologic systems perturbed by COVID-19, HMB may represent a useful support for older patients suffering from long-term COVID-19 sequelae.

Tricarboxylic Acid Cycle Intermediates

Malic acid, citric acid, and succinic acid are TCA cycle intermediates with a well-established role in mitochondrial energy metabolism. Once considered byproducts of cellular metabolism to be used for the biosynthesis of macromolecules (eg, lipids, nucleotides, proteins), TCA cycle intermediates are now recognized as important mitochondrial signaling molecules regulating multiple cellular functions.[46] Indeed, TCA cycle metabolites may also modulate chromatin remodeling, DNA methylation, posttranslational protein modifications, platelet activity, and immunity.[15,47,48]

Supplementation with TCA cycle intermediates may help preserve mitochondrial biogenesis and function and fulfill the increased metabolic demands of older people recovering from COVID-19. In this context, TCA cycle metabolites may support the beneficial effects of amino acid supplementation in the prevention of mitochondrial dysfunction, oxidative damage, and muscle loss.[49] Novel formulas combining mixtures of amino acids plus TCA intermediates, such as citric, succinic, and malic acid, and B group vitamins, were tested for their effects on mitochondrial bioenergetics and antioxidant response both in vitro and in animal models of aging.[50,51] In murine neural stem cells and human-induced pluripotent stem cells, mitochondrial function, oxidant scavenging mechanisms, and neuronal stem cells differentiation were boosted via activation of the mechanistic target of rapamycin complex 1 and nuclear factor erythroid 2 like 2 (Nrf2)-mediated gene expression.[50] In a mouse model of accelerated muscular and cognitive aging, the combination of amino acids plus TCA cycle metabolites and cofactors preserved mitochondrial efficiency, muscle mass, and physical and cognitive abilities by acting on proliferator-activated receptor γ coactivator 1α and NRF2 in skeletal muscle and hippocampus.[51]

Further investigation is warranted to evaluate the potential effects of TCA cycle metabolites (alone or combined with other nutrients) to contrast long-term consequences of COVID-19.

Micronutrients

Nutritional surveys indicate that vitamin and mineral deficiencies are highly prevalent in older adults. Micronutrient deficiencies are associated with increased risk of noncommunicable diseases, such as fatigue, cardiometabolic disease, musculoskeletal disorders, and cognitive impairment.[52] Micronutrients, including selenium, iron, zinc, and magnesium, are also critical for the proper functioning of the immune system.[53]

Selenium

Selenium is an essential trace element and is mainly present in the form of selenoproteins. Selenium is involved in several physiologic processes, including neurologic, endocrinologic, cardiovascular, and immune functions.[54]

Several studies have investigated the role of selenium in modulating the immune response, and for this reason, a putative role for selenium has been evoked in the context of COVID-19.[55] Evidence in human, animal, and cellular models suggests that selenium plays an important role in response to viral infections, including respiratory viruses,[56] while its deficiency seems to increase host susceptibility to infections.[55,57] In viral infections, selenoproteins inhibit type I interferon responses and viral transcriptional activators.[54,55] Selenium supplementation stimulates innate immune system and increases CD4+ T cells and natural killer cell response.[58] Selenium also modulates the secretion of proinflammatory interleukins by inhibiting nuclear factor κB (NF-κB).[55] Selenium deficiency has been correlated to greater secretion of interleukin-6 (IL-6) in older adults,[59] whereas higher levels of selenium are associated with reduced C-reactive protein (CRP) circulating levels.[60] Low plasma concentration of selenium was also correlated with increased tissue damage and organ failure, prothrombotic activity, and overall mortality in patients in intensive care, which could explain a correlation with severity of symptoms in patients with COVID-19 and possible COVID-19 sequelae in long haulers.[3,61–63] Several studies have reported that circulating selenium concentrations were lower in patients with COVID-19 as compared with healthy controls and associated with COVID-19 severity and mortality.[64,65]

Low selenium levels may increase individual susceptibility to SARS-CoV-2 infection, influence the severity of the disease,[66,67] and be related to postacute sequelae and long-lasting symptoms.[68]

Iron

Iron is essential for all living organisms, being a crucial component of hundreds of proteins involved in fundamental biological processes, including oxygen transport, energy production, and nucleic acid synthesis.[69] During viral infections, the rapid viral proliferation determines a competition for iron between the invading pathogen and the host.[70] Moreover, iron homeostasis influences both the innate and the adaptive host immune response. In fact, hypoferremia is linked to altered B- and T-lymphocyte proliferation and function[71] and is associated with higher levels of proinflammatory cytokines and reactive oxygen species.[72] Low-iron levels have been associated with the severity of respiratory insufficiency, acute multiorgan failure, and mortality in patients with COVID-19.[73–75] Iron status parameters, such as ferritin, transferrin, and hepcidin, which respectively serve to store, transport, and absorb iron in the human body, may be considered risk factors and clinical biomarkers for COVID-19 prognosis.[76] In particular, meta-analyses have correlated high-ferritin levels with COVID-19 severity and mortality.[77–79] Ferritin stimulates the expression of proinflammatory cytokines, such as IL-1β, IL-6, IL-12, and tumor necrosis factor-α (TNF-α),[71] and a gradual reduction of its circulating levels has been demonstrated in patients with COVID-19 after infusion of monoclonal antibodies targeting IL-6 receptor.[200] Preliminary data from a prospective observational cohort study in patients with mild to critical COVID-19 show that alterations in iron homeostasis may persist for at least 2 months after acute infection and are associated with nonresolving lung disorders and impaired physical performance.[80] Iron deficiency was associated with elevated levels of inflammation markers, such as IL-6 and CRP.[80] Finally, low-iron levels could theoretically impair the efficacy of COVID-19 vaccination,[71] underlining the importance of monitoring iron levels, especially in older adults with long COVID.

Based on the available evidence, iron supplementation, especially in older adults with low iron and hemoglobin levels, could be particularly useful for reducing the level of inflammation, mitigating persistent symptoms (such as fatigue and dyspnea), and improving immune response to vaccination.

Zinc

Zinc is the second most abundant trace metal in the human body after iron and is essential for the maintenance of immune health, cell homeostasis, and reproduction.[81,82] Zinc deficiency is quite common in the general population and is also associated with immune dysfunction, affecting both the innate and the adaptive immune systems.[83,84] Inadequate zinc intake has been associated with increased risk of upper- and lower-respiratory tract infections, especially in older adults,[85,86] whereas supplementation with zinc gluconate seems to reduce duration and severity of common cold symptoms.[87]

Zinc may inhibit coronavirus RNA polymerase activity in vitro and viral replication in cultured cells.[88] Zinc has also an immunomodulatory, antioxidant, and anti-inflammatory role that could influence the trajectory of SARS-CoV-2 infection, and its supplementation could ameliorate lung function, enhance mucociliary clearance, and reduce ventilator-induced lung injury in critical patients with COVID-19.[85] Lower serum zinc levels were found in patients with severe COVID-19 with acute respiratory distress syndrome and associated with a higher rate of complications and in-hospital length of stay.[64,85] Zinc deficiency could also be connected to the onset and persistence of symptoms such as anosmia and dysgeusia, which can last for a variable amount of time after resolution of acute infection.[89]

Zinc supplementation was tested for its potential role in contrasting the consequences of SARS-CoV-2 infection. However, available data on the efficacy of zinc supplementation for the management of patients with COVID-19 are scarce and contradictory.[64,90,91] A prospective randomized clinical trial, COVID A to Z study, evaluated the efficacy of a treatment with zinc gluconate, ascorbic acid, or their combination in shortening the duration of COVID-19 symptoms.[92] The study failed to demonstrate a significant improvement in symptoms, and the study was stopped for futility.

Further studies are needed to evaluate the effects of zinc or mixtures of micronutrients, including zinc in both acute COVID-19 and in long COVID-19 syndrome.

Magnesium

Magnesium is essential for several physiologic functions and biochemical reactions and may exert important anti-inflammatory and antioxidant functions.[93,94]

Although severe magnesium deficiency with clinical symptoms is quite rare, hypomagnesemia is frequent in patients in the intensive care unit, regardless of the cause of admission, and is associated with increased mortality, higher need for ventilator support and incidence of sepsis, and longer hospital stays.[95] Although there are no significant data on magnesium homeostasis in patients with COVID-19, it has been suggested that magnesium deficiency could modulate the progress and severity of SARS-CoV-2 infection.[96] Magnesium supplementation protects organs and tissues from damage through multiple mechanisms and could potentially influence the natural history of COVID-19.[96]

It is well known that magnesium exerts anticholinergic, antihistaminic, and anti-inflammatory activities, reduces the risk of airway hyperreactivity and wheezing, and promotes bronchodilation by inhibiting bronchial smooth muscle contraction via blockage of calcium channels.[94,97] A systematic review demonstrated that a single infusion of 1.2 or 2 g of magnesium sulfate in adults with exacerbations of asthma was associated with a reduction in hospitalization rate and improved lung function in patients who did not respond to standard treatment (ie, oxygen, nebulized short-acting β2-agonist, and intravenous corticosteroids).[98] In addition, magnesium reduces the secretion of transforming growth factor β1, thereby preventing lung fibrosis,[99] a rare but fearsome consequence of COVID-19.

Magnesium plays a role in modulating the innate and adaptive immune system.[93,94] Subclinical magnesium deficiency is correlated with low-grade chronic inflammation, which can be crucial for the prognosis of COVID-19 and the persistence of COVID-19 symptoms.[93] It has been demonstrated that magnesium sulfate supplementation downregulates inflammatory response and oxidative stress by inhibiting chemokine and cytokines, such as IL-1, IL-6, IL-8, TNF-α, and CRP, which are often significantly elevated in severe COVID-19 cases.[93,94] Magnesium may also modulate the adaptive immune system, influencing the proliferation and the activation of $CD4^+$ and $CD8^+$ T lymphocytes.[96] Furthermore, magnesium exerts an important role in maintaining endothelial function and vascular integrity.[100] In response to an acute inflammation stimulus, such as SARS-CoV-2 infection, the endothelium increases the secretion of prothrombotic factors. Accumulating evidence suggests that the endothelium might be directly affected in patients with COVID-19.[101] Magnesium supplementation, especially in older adults, could help prevent the risk of thromboembolism in COVID-19 and long-term consequences in COVID-19 survivors.[102] In critically ill patients with COVID-19, magnesium sulfate supplementation can represent a supportive treatment with promising beneficial effects.[94] A retrospective observational study demonstrated that in hospitalized patients with COVID-19 aged 50 years and older, a combination of oral vitamin D3, magnesium, and vitamin B12 supplementation for up to 14 days significantly reduced the need of oxygen therapy compared with controls.[103]

Despite the lack of clinical trials and well-powered studies in patients with COVID-19, magnesium supplementation seems to find a potential application in controlling respiratory symptoms, but also in modulating inflammation, cardiovascular and neurologic disorders, and electrolyte abnormalities. The monitoring of magnesium status should be encouraged, as it may influence immune homeostasis and help decrease morbidity and mortality in patients with COVID-19.[93]

Bromelain

Bromelain is a proteolytic enzyme derived from the fruit and stem of pineapple. Bromelain is commonly used as an anti-inflammatory agent, although its potential biological activity spans from respiratory, digestive, immune, and circulatory systems to anticancer and antimicrobial therapy.[104]

Bromelain regulates inflammatory processes through the modulation of NF-κB and cyclooxygenase 2 pathways that regulate the synthesis of inflammatory cytokines and prostaglandin E2 and thromboxane A2, respectively.[105] Moreover, bromelain has fibrinolytic and antithrombotic properties[106,107] and may also exert analgesic effects by regulating the synthesis of pain mediators, such as bradykinin.[108] The decrease in bradykinin levels induced by bromelain may also indirectly act on inflammatory response through the regulation of vascular permeability and reduction in edema. Bromelain showed immunomodulatory effects both in vitro and in vivo.[109] Bromelain may simultaneously enhance and inhibit T-cell responses by acting on accessory cells and directly on T cells. Moreover, bromelain enhanced T-cell–dependent, antigen-specific, B-cell antibody responses in vivo.[109]

In vitro studies suggest that bromelain may also inhibit SARS-CoV-2 infection by targeting ACE-2, transmembrane serine protease 2, and SARS-CoV-2 S-protein.[110]

Considering its multiple potential activities on mechanisms involved in acute and chronic COVID-19 phases, bromelain could represent a candidate therapeutic agent for the management of COVID-19. In this context, bromelain may also increase the absorption of curcumin and other bioactive compounds with possible anti–COVID-19 activities after oral administration.[111] Currently, data about the properties of bromelain on persistent symptoms related to long COVID-19 are lacking, but it can be hypothesized that its biological activities might help in the process of recovery from chronic fatigue, joint pain, and myalgia.[104]

Troxerutin

Troxerutin is a flavonoid derived from rutin that can be found in tea, coffee, cereals, fruits, and vegetables. Troxerutin exerts multiple biological functions, including antioxidant, anti-inflammatory, nephroprotective, antithrombotic, antidiabetic, and neuroprotective effects.[112] Following ingestion, flavonoids are partially digested by microbiome, which facilitates the absorption by small or large bowel.

Troxerutin exerts its antioxidant functions through direct free radical scavenging activity[113] and by enhancing the activity of glutathione and antioxidant enzymes, such as superoxide dismutase, catalase, and glutathione peroxidase.[114] Through its antioxidant activities, troxerutin might preserve epithelial cells, fibroblasts, and lymphocytes from oxidative stress-induced apoptosis.[113]

Troxerutin was found to protect against gentamycin-induced acute kidney injury in rats through the downregulation of inflammatory cytokines (IL-10, TNF-α, and IL-6), the reduction of apoptotic cell death, and the induction of renal tissue regenerative capacity, by acting on p38 mitogen-activated protein kinase signaling.[115]

Troxerutin protects the hippocampus against amyloid-beta induced oxidative stress and apoptosis by reducing the acetylcholinesterase activity and oxidative stress.[114] In a rat model of traumatic brain injury, troxerutin exerted multiple protective effects through the regulation of endothelial NOS activity.[116] Moreover, troxerutin demonstrated anxiolytic- and antidepressant-like activities in rodents.[117]

In rat models of type 1 and type 2 diabetes, troxerutin preserved male fertility and protected against diabetic cardiomyopathy through the reduction of reactive oxygen species and its activity of NF-κB, serine/threonine kinase 1, and insulin receptor substrate 1.[118,119]

Data on the activity of troxerutin in COVID-19 are currently lacking. However, its antioxidant and anti-inflammatory properties might be helpful for both the acute and the chronic consequences of SARS-CoV-2 infection.

Lactoferrin

Lactoferrin is an iron-binding glycoprotein, which acts as a host defense molecule against microbes. Lactoferrin is mainly secreted from exocrine glands and is present in granules in neutrophils following infections.[120] Lactoferrin prevents microbial and viral adhesion to human cells through its iron-chelating ability, which reduces availability of iron used for microbial growth, aggregation, and biofilm formation.[121] The activity of lactoferrin is mostly bacteriostatic, but a lethal effect has been demonstrated. One of its derivates, lactoferricin, tends to inactivate the lipid A from lipopolysaccharide of gram-negative bacteria. Lactoferrin may also have a bactericidal effect on gram-positive bacteria. Lactoferrin exerts its antiviral activity through different mechanisms at the mucosal level, including binding to heparan sulfate glycosaminoglycans, viral particles, and viral receptors, thus limiting viral entry.[122]

In vitro, bovine lactoferrin blocks human cell apoptosis induced by influenza A virus.[123] In vitro and in vivo studies showed that lactoferrin may also inhibit cytomegalovirus[124] and herpes simplex virus infection.[125] The antiviral activity of lactoferrin has been demonstrated against a multitude of viruses, including respiratory syncytial virus, poliovirus, hepatitis B virus, hepatitis C virus, alphaviruses, hantavirus, human papillomavirus, adenovirus, and enterovirus.[126] Given its immunomodulatory and antiviral properties, the use of lactoferrin was also proposed to contrast SARS-CoV-2 infection.[127] In vitro and in silico assays showed that lactoferrin may have an antiviral activity against SARS-CoV-2 through direct attachment to both SARS-CoV-2 spike S glycoprotein and cell surface components.[128] Lactoferrin may also modulate the inflammatory cascade through the reduction of IL-6, TNF-α, and ferritin levels.[129] A preliminary study testing the antiviral effect of oral and intranasal liposomal bovine lactoferrin in asymptomatic and patients with mild to moderate COVID-19 showed that lactoferrin treatment induced fast symptom resolution compared with standard care.[130] Treatment with lactoferrin also elicited a significant decrease in serum ferritin, IL-6, and D-dimer.

Based on available evidence, lactoferrin may represent a promising molecule to be used in both patients with acute COVID-19 or patients with postacute COVID-19 syndrome. Further investigations are needed to corroborate the positive preliminary findings obtained in patients with COVID-19, and to determine whether lactoferrin supplementation alone or with other bioactive compounds may result in additive beneficial effects against acute and postacute COVID-19.

Probiotics

The gastrointestinal system may be affected during acute and postacute COVID-19.[131] Gastrointestinal symptoms, such as diarrhea, nausea, vomiting, and loss of appetite, are commonly experienced by people with COVID-19. SARS-CoV-2 RNA may be detected in stools even after viral clearance in the respiratory tract.[132] Moreover, alterations in gut microbiota were associated with COVID-19 severity, possibly as a consequence of a "leaky gut" phenomenon and the release of microbial products and toxins into systemic circulation.[133,134] Long-term antibiotic therapies, hospitalization, stress, comorbidities, and the direct action of SARS-CoV-2 on ACE2 receptor at the gastrointestinal level are associated with gut dysbiosis. Perturbations in gut microbiota may persist months after acute COVID-19 and may be associated with long-term complications.[135]

Probiotics are "live microbes that, when administered in adequate amounts, confer health benefits on their hosts."[136] Probiotics (mainly Bifidobacteria and Lactobacilli) may exert relevant immunomodulatory functions on the gut-lung axis.[137] Probiotics increase host mucosal defense through the stimulation of immunoglobulin A secretion, induce polarization of the immune response toward Th1, modulate cytokine production, and produce metabolites, such as short chain fatty acids, that contribute to set the tone of the immune system.[138] Probiotics may have also anti-inflammatory,[139] antioxidant,[140] and antiviral properties.[141] Interestingly, an in silico molecular docking approach suggested that metabolites from *Lactobacillus plantarum* may have potential antiviral activity against SARS-CoV-2 by targeting helicase nsp13.[142] Probiotics may also have synergistic antiviral activities when combined with compounds with antimicrobial properties. For instance, Lacticaseibacillus paracasei DG strain enhances the lactoferrin anti–SARS-CoV-2 response in Caco-2 cells.[143]

Numerous studies are currently testing the use of different mixtures of probiotics as adjunctive treatment for the management of both acute and postacute COVID-19.[141,144,145] Preliminary evidence suggests that probiotics administration may reduce secondary infections in people with severe COVID-19.[146] The consumption of a specific bacterial formulation containing strains of *Streptococcus thermophilus, Lactobacillus acidophilus, Lactobacillus helveticus, Lactobacillus paracasei, L plantarum, Lactobacillus brevis*, and *Bifidobacterium lactis* was associated with remission of gastrointestinal symptoms and reduced risk of respiratory failure in hospitalized patients with COVID-19.[145] In COVID-19 outpatients, the administration of a mixture of

Lactiplantibacillus plantarum and *Pediococcus acidilactici* strains improved viral clearance and reduced both respiratory and gastrointestinal symptoms compared with placebo.[147]

Further studies are needed to assess the effects of specific probiotic formulations and/or the combination of probiotics with other bioactive compounds on long-term COVID-19 sequelae.

The use of probiotics may be particularly recommended in older patients with COVID-19, in whom age-related factors, including frailty, multimorbidity, and malnutrition, may aggravate gut dysbiosis.

Vitamin D

Vitamin D plays a crucial role in the regulation of calcium and bone metabolism.[148] Accumulating evidence from preclinical and observational studies suggests that vitamin D could be involved in many extraskeletal pathways, including immune and muscle function, reproduction, and energy metabolism.[148] Vitamin D may modulate different aspects of the innate and adaptive immune response.[149] Both vitamin D receptor and enzymes involved in vitamin D metabolism are expressed by several immune cell types, including lymphocytes, monocytes, macrophages, and dendritic cells.[149]

Vitamin D may support innate immunity by stimulating the synthesis of several antimicrobial peptides, including cathelicidins and defensivins.[150] Vitamin D may also regulate the activity of antigen-presenting cells, T- and B-cell differentiation, and the balance between proinflammatory and anti-inflammatory cytokines.[151] Low vitamin D levels were associated with increased risk of numerous immune-related conditions, including type 1 diabetes,[152] multiple sclerosis,[153] and rheumatoid arthritis.[154] Furthermore, people with vitamin D deficiency tend to be more prone to develop acute respiratory infections.[155]

Vitamin D deficiency has been associated with increased risk of SARS-CoV-2 infection and worse clinical outcomes, including more severe lung impairment, need for respiratory support and intensive care, and mortality.[156,157] Hence, vitamin D supplementation has been tested as a candidate adjunctive treatment for COVID-19. In asymptomatic or mildly symptomatic individuals with SARS-CoV-2 and vitamin D deficiency, a 7-day administration of high-dose vitamin D (60,000 IU of cholecalciferol per day) accelerated viral clearance compared with placebo.[158] Vitamin D supplementation taken before or during COVID-19 was associated with better 3-month survival in older adults hospitalized for COVID-19 compared with nonsupplemented peers.[159] However, a recent living systematic review found insufficient evidence to determine the benefits of vitamin D supplementation as a treatment of COVID-19, owing to the heterogeneity of studies, including different supplementation strategies, formulations, vitamin D status of participants, and reported outcomes.[160]

As for postacute COVID-19, data on the association between vitamin D levels and the persistence of symptoms are scarce. In a small group of COVID-19 survivors from Dublin, persistent fatigue and reduced exercise tolerance were not associated with vitamin D levels.[161]

Because of the multiple effects of vitamin D on biological pathways associated with long COVID and its relevance for the overall health status, vitamin D supplementation should be considered to avoid the detrimental consequences of vitamin deficiency. This holds true in particular for vulnerable people, such as older COVID-19 survivors, in whom vitamin D may also contrast geriatric conditions, such as frailty and sarcopenia, that are associated with negative health outcomes and may further reduce the quality of life.[162]

Pollen-Based Herbal Extracts

Pollen, the male gametophyte of the flower, has long been used for therapeutic purposes by various ancient civilizations.[163] Pollen contains a mixture of amino acids, carbohydrates, minerals, and bioactive substances that vary depending on the plant source and geographic origin, climatic conditions, soil type, and the activity of bees.[164]

Purified cytoplasm of pollen (PCP) is a nonhormonal herbal remedy used to manage vasomotor symptoms and sleep and mood disorders in menopausal women.[165] Even if the mechanisms of action of PCP are not fully understood, this compound seems to act as a selective serotonin reuptake inhibitor (SSRI)-like agent to increase serotonin availability in hypothalamic serotonergic neurons. This explains, at least partly, its efficacy in controlling thermoregulation, and sleep and mood disorders in menopausal woman, without the adverse effects of currently prescribed SSRIs.[166] Another putative mechanism action of PCP could be based on the precursors of serotonin. Indeed, tryptophan and methyl serotonins have been identified in low concentrations in PCP extracts, even if their contribution to intraneuronal serotonin synthesis could be negligible.[166] Studies conducted in women with symptomatic menopause demonstrated that PCP supplementation improved sleep quality and quality of life and reduced hot flushes, fatigue, and muscle and joint pain.[165,167] The most common symptoms complained of by COVID-19 long haulers are fatigue, muscle weakness, and sleep difficulties, with a higher risk of developing anxiety or depression. Given the accumulating evidence on the effects of PCP in contrasting these symptoms in menopausal women, it could be speculated that PCP may be used as a remedy to mitigate persisting symptoms in long COVID patients.

Beetroot Juice

Beetroot juice, which is obtained from the red beetroot (*Beta vulgaris*), has spurred much attention owing to its potential beneficial effects on cardiovascular health, metabolic homeostasis, inflammation, and pulmonary function.[168–170] The multiple health benefits of beetroot juice have traditionally been attributed to its high nitrate (NO_3^-) content. Following ingestion, beetroot juice (as well as other nitrate-rich foods, such as leafy green vegetables) increases NO availability through the nitrate-nitrite-NO pathway.[171] Dietary nitrate administration in the form of beetroot juice has been extensively studied in sport nutrition, owing to its purported beneficial effects on physical performance.[172] In this context, beetroot juice may improve both endurance and power exercise performance through increasing NO bioavailability, which in turn modulates mitochondrial respiration, reduces oxygen cost of exercise, and improves muscular and cerebral perfusion.[173,174] Recent evidence has shown that the stimulation of the nitrate-nitrite-NO pathway by beetroot juice consumption may improve endothelial function, as measured by flow-mediated dilation, in persons with or at risk of endothelial dysfunction, including older adults,[175] people with peripheral artery disease,[176] pregnant women,[177] and persons with hypercholesterolemia[178] and hypertension.[179] Moreover, beetroot juice ingestion was associated with a reduction in blood pressure in normotensive[180] and hypertensive people,[181] and in older adults.[182] Interestingly, higher baseline blood pressure, being overweight or obese, and male sex were associated with better response to beetroot juice supplementation.[183] Beetroot juice consumption may also increase NO bioavailability in upper and lower airways, which boosts innate immune defense and protects against respiratory tract infections.[184] In people with chronic obstructive pulmonary disease, nitrate-rich beetroot juice improves exercise tolerance as measured by the Borg Rating of Perceived Exertion scale.[185]

Accumulating evidence in preclinical models of inflammatory diseases suggests that inorganic nitrate and nitrite may modulate the inflammatory response by acting on neutrophil and monocyte/macrophage recruitment and activation.[171] Only a few studies have investigated the effects of beetroot juice ingestion on the inflammatory response in humans. In healthy older volunteers and individuals with hypercholesterolemia, both acute and medium-term supplementation with beetroot juice was associated with a reduction in proinflammatory monocyte-platelets aggregates.[178,186] Moreover, a decrease in neutrophil activation was observed within 3 hours of beetroot juice supplementation.[186]

Besides nitrate, beetroot juice also contains a plethora of bioactive ingredients with antioxidant and anti-inflammatory properties, including polyphenols, carotenoids, betalains, and organic acids.[169,187] In particular, betalains, a class of natural pigments that includes the red-violet betacyanins and the yellow-orange betaxanthins,[188] have gained much attention owing to their ability of stimulating the activity of antioxidant enzymes and inhibiting the inflammatory cascade.[169,187] Betanin, the most abundant betalain found in beetroots, may directly scavenge reactive oxygen species[189] and increase the expression of catalase, superoxide dismutase, and glutathione peroxidase through the activation of Nrf2/antioxidant response element pathway.[190] Moreover, betanin and its derivatives may exert anti-inflammatory effects through the inhibition of COX2[191] and lipoxygenase 1.[192] Betanin may also inhibit NF-κB, a master regulator of the inflammatory response.[193] Very few studies have investigated the anti-inflammatory effect of betanins in humans.[194] Ten-day supplementation with betalain-rich beetroot extracts reduced the concentration of TNF-α and IL-6 in people with osteoarthritis.[195] Consumption of both raw beetroot juice and cooked beets reduced intracellular adhesion molecule-1, vascular endothelial adhesion molecule-1, CRP, IL-6, E-selectin, and TNF-α in adults with hypertension.[181] Although both supplementation forms were effective, people consuming beetroot juice showed greater improvement in systemic inflammatory parameters, as well as in blood pressure and endothelial function.[181] Collectively, these findings suggest that beetroot juice may have multiple beneficial effects on crucial physiologic functions that could be exploited against COVID-19 and its systemic consequences.[196]

Further studies are needed to investigate the effects of supplementation with beetroot juice and/or its derivatives in patients with COVID-19 across disease stages and during recovery.

Ongoing Studies

Based on the putative beneficial effects against several processes involved in long COVID, a panel of bioactive foods, nutraceuticals, and supplements is being tested in the outpatient service at the Fondazione Policlinico A. Gemelli IRCSS (Rome, Italy) **(Fig. 1)**

A combination of amino acids and malic, succinic, and citric acid (Amino-Ther Pro; Professional Dietetics, Milan, Italy) has been tested in patients with long COVID with malnutrition and fatigue. Preliminary data on the first 20 patients show improvement in nutritional status and better performance on the handgrip strength and five-repetition chair-stand test after 2 months of treatment (The Gemelli Against COVID-19 Post-Acute Care Study Group, 2022).

In a second pilot study, patients with persistent fatigue received a combination of amino acids and micronutrients (including magnesium, selenium, iron) (ApportAl; PharmaNutra, Pisa, Italy). After 6 weeks of treatment, muscle mass and strength improved with a significant reduction of inflammatory markers (CRP and IL-6) (The Gemelli Against COVID-19 Post-Acute Care Study Group, 2022).

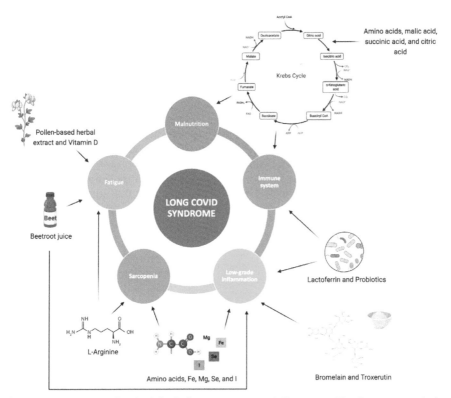

Fig. 1. Long COVID pathophysiological processes potentially targeted by the nutraceuticals and dietary supplements described in the study.

L-Arginine plus vitamin C (Bioarginina C; Farmaceutici Damor, Naples, Italy) has been tested in COVID-19 survivors with persistent fatigue. Preliminary results on the first 46 patients treated with Bioarginina C indicate reduction in fatigue, better physical performance, and better quality of life (The Gemelli Against COVID-19 Post-Acute Care Study Group, 2022).

A combination of bromelain and troxerutin (BromeREX; Pharma G, Anzio, Italy) has been tested in patients with long COVID with increased inflammation. In the first 20 participants treated with bromelain and troxerutin, attenuation of post–COVID-19 symptoms and significant reduction of serum CRP levels were observed (The Gemelli Against COVID-19 Post-Acute Care Study Group, 2022).

A combination of lactoferrin and *L paracasei* (Pirv-F20; Farmagens Health Care, Rome, Italy) has been administered to persons with long COVID. Preliminary data suggest a significant reduction in inflammatory status and improvement in fatigue, dyspnea, and joint and muscle pain (The Gemelli Against COVID-19 Post-Acute Care Study Group, 2022).

A pollen-based herbal extract (Femal; Shionogi, Milan, Italy) has been prescribed to women with persistent fatigue, sleep disorders, and cognitive distress (brain fog) following an acute COVID-19 episode. A substantial improvement in persistent symptoms and quality has been observed (The Gemelli Against COVID-19 Post-Acute Care Study Group, 2022).

A beetroot juice (Aureli Mario S.S. Agricola, Ortucchio, Italy) with a well-characterized phytochemical profile[197] has been tested in COVID-19 survivors with fatigue. Changes in physical performance (6-minute walking test, handgrip strength), endothelial function, inflammatory status, urinary and fecal metabolomics, and metagenomics are being evaluated. Preliminary data suggest that beetroot juice supplementation induces favorable immune and metabolic changes (The Gemelli Against COVID-19 Post-Acute Care Study Group, 2022).

Results from the authors' ongoing studies may indicate novel strategies for the management of long COVID as part of multimodal interventions. An example of such interventions combining personalized nutrition counseling and physical activity was successfully in the Sarcopenia and Physical fRailty IN older people: multi-componenT Treatment strategies" (SPRINTT) project.[198] A multimodel intervention inspired by SPRINTT is currently being implemented at the authors' outpatient clinic.[199]

SUMMARY

Long COVID affects a large share of persons of all age groups but may be especially burdensome for vulnerable older adults. Long COVID has a complex pathophysiology encompassing inflammatory and autoimmune processes, perturbations in metabolic pathways, and alterations in endothelial function and redox homeostasis.

The management of long COVID requires a multidimensional approach that should include a comprehensive nutritional assessment. Several food bioactive compounds, nutraceuticals, and supplements may target specific pathways involved in long COVID and may, therefore, be used as an adjunctive therapy to manage the condition.

CLINICS CARE POINTS

- Long COVID affects a large share of persons of all age groups but may be especially burdensome for vulnerable older adults.
- Long COVID has a complex pathophysiology, and its management requires a multidimensional approach that should include a nutritional assessment.
- Food bioactive compounds and nutraceuticals may target specific pathways involved in long COVID.

DISCLOSURE

Unconditional support to research activities at the postacute outpatient service, Fondazione Policlinico Universitario Agostino Gemelli IRCCS (Rome, Italy), was provided by Professional Dietetics, PharmaNutra, Farmaceutici Damor, Pharma G, Farmagens Health Care, Shionogi, Aureli Mario S.S. Agricola. The study was also supported by Ministero della Salute - Ricerca Corrente 2022. The funders had no role in the writing of the article nor decision to submit the article for publication.

ACKNOWLEDGMENTS

The author is grateful to thank "The Gemelli Against COVID-19 Post-Acute Care Study Group".The gemelli against COVID-19 postacute care study group is composed as follows: *Steering committee*: Landi Francesco, Gremese Elisa. *Coordination*: Bernabei

Roberto, Fantoni Massimo, Gasbarrini Antonio. Field Investigators: Gastroenterology team: Settanni Carlo Romano. Geriatric team: Benvenuto Francesca, Bramato Giulia, Brandi Vincenzo, Carfi Angelo, Ciciarello Francesca, Lo Monaco Maria Rita, Martone Anna Maria, Marzetti Emanuele, Napolitano Carmen, Pagano Francesco, Rocchi Sara, Rota Elisabetta, Salerno Andrea, Tosato Matteo, Tritto Marcello, Calvani Riccardo, Catalano Lucio, Picca Anna, Savera Giulia. Infectious disease team: Cauda Roberto, Tamburrini Enrica, Borghetti A, Di Gianbenedetto Simona, Murri Rita, Cingolani Antonella, Ventura Giulio, Taddei E, Moschese D, Ciccullo A. Internal Medicine team: Stella Leonardo, Addolorato Giovanni, Franceschi Francesco, Mingrone Gertrude, Zocco MA. Microbiology team: Sanguinetti Maurizio, Cattani Paola, Marchetti Simona, Posteraro Brunella, Sali M. Neurology team: Bizzarro Alessandra, Lauria Alessandra. Ophthalmology team: Rizzo Stanislao, Savastano Maria Cristina, Gambini G, Cozzupoli GM, Culiersi C. Otolaryngology team: Passali Giulio Cesare, Paludetti Gaetano, Galli Jacopo, Crudo F, Di Cintio G, Longobardi Y, Tricarico L, Santantonio M. Pediatric team: Buonsenso Danilo, Valentini P, Pata D, Sinatti D, De Rose C. Pneumology team: Richeldi Luca, Lombardi Francesco, Calabrese A. Psychiatric team: Sani Gabriele, Janiri Delfina, Giuseppin G, Molinaro M, Modica M. Radiology team: Natale Luigi, Larici Anna Rita, Marano Riccardo. Rheumatology team: Paglionico Annamaria, Petricca Luca, Gigante Luca, Natalello G, Fedele AL, Lizzio MM, Tolusso B, Alivernini S. Vascular team: Santoliquido Angelo, Santoro Luca, Nesci A, Popolla V.

REFERENCES

1. Gupta A, Madhavan MV, Sehgal K, et al. Extrapulmonary manifestations of COVID-19. Nat Med 2020;26(7):1017–32.
2. Report of the WHO-China joint mission on coronavirus disease 2019 (COVID-19). Available at: https://www.who.int/docs/default-source/coronaviruse/who-china-joint-mission-on-covid-19-final-report. Accessed April 13, 2022.
3. Nalbandian A, Sehgal K, Gupta A, et al. Post-acute COVID-19 syndrome. Nat Med 2021;27(4):601–15.
4. Mehandru S, Merad M. Pathological sequelae of long-haul COVID. Nat Immunol 2022;23(2):194–202.
5. Groff D, Sun A, Ssentongo AE, et al. Short-term and long-term rates of postacute sequelae of SARS-CoV-2 infection: a systematic review. JAMA Netw Open 2021; 4(10). https://doi.org/10.1001/JAMANETWORKOPEN.2021.28568.
6. Bliddal S, Banasik K, Pedersen OB, et al. Acute and persistent symptoms in non-hospitalized PCR-confirmed COVID-19 patients. Sci Rep 2021;11(1). https://doi.org/10.1038/S41598-021-92045-X.
7. Tosato M, Carfi A, Martis I, et al. Prevalence and predictors of persistence of COVID-19 symptoms in older adults: a single-center study. J Am Med Dir Assoc 2021;22(9):1840–4.
8. Merad M, Blish CA, Sallusto F, et al. The immunology and immunopathology of COVID-19. Science 2022;375(6585):1122–7.
9. Douaud G, Lee S, Alfaro-Almagro F, et al. SARS-CoV-2 is associated with changes in brain structure in UK Biobank. Nature 2022. https://doi.org/10.1038/S41586-022-04569-5.
10. Mongelli A, Barbi V, Zamperla MG, et al. Evidence for biological age acceleration and telomere shortening in COVID-19 survivors. Int J Mol Sci 2021;22(11). https://doi.org/10.3390/IJMS22116151.
11. Bartleson JM, Radenkovic D, Covarrubias AJ, et al. SARS-CoV-2, COVID-19 and the ageing immune system. Nat Aging 2021;1(9):769–82.

12. Ghidoli M, Colombo F, Sangiorgio S, et al. Food containing bioactive flavonoids and other phenolic or sulfur phytochemicals with antiviral effect: can we design a promising diet against COVID-19? Front Nutr 2021;8. https://doi.org/10.3389/FNUT.2021.661331.

13. Galanakis CM, Aldawoud TMS, Rizou M, et al. Food ingredients and active compounds against the coronavirus disease (COVID-19) pandemic: a comprehensive review. Foods 2020;9(11). https://doi.org/10.3390/FOODS9111701.

14. Landi F, Gremese E, Bernabei R, et al. Post-COVID-19 global health strategies: the need for an interdisciplinary approach. Aging Clin Exp Res 2020;32(8): 1613–20.

15. Kelly B, Pearce EL. Amino assets: how amino acids support immunity. Cell Metab 2020;32(2):154–75.

16. Newsholme P, Curi R, Pithon Curi TC, et al. Glutamine metabolism by lymphocytes, macrophages, and neutrophils: its importance in health and disease. J Nutr Biochem 1999;10(6):316–24.

17. Palmieri EM, Gonzalez-Cotto M, Baseler WA, et al. Nitric oxide orchestrates metabolic rewiring in M1 macrophages by targeting aconitase 2 and pyruvate dehydrogenase. Nat Commun 2020;11(1). https://doi.org/10.1038/S41467-020-14433-7.

18. Lam WY, Jash A, Yao CH, et al. Metabolic and transcriptional modules independently diversify plasma cell lifespan and function. Cell Rep 2018;24(9):2479–92. https://doi.org/10.1016/J.CELREP.2018.07.084, e6.

19. Cruzat V, Rogero MM, Keane KN, et al. Glutamine: metabolism and immune function, supplementation and clinical translation. Nutrients 2018;10(11). https://doi.org/10.3390/NU10111564.

20. Nie C, He T, Zhang W, et al. Branched chain amino acids: beyond nutrition metabolism. Int J Mol Sci 2018;19(4). https://doi.org/10.3390/IJMS19040954.

21. Calder PC. Branched-chain amino acids and immunity. J Nutr 2006;136(1 Suppl). https://doi.org/10.1093/JN/136.1.288S.

22. Ma N, Guo P, Zhang J, et al. Nutrients mediate intestinal bacteria-mucosal immune crosstalk. Front Immunol 2018;9(JAN). https://doi.org/10.3389/FIMMU.2018.00005.

23. Adebayo A, Varzideh F, Wilson S, et al. l-Arginine and COVID-19: an Update. Nutrients 2021;13(11). https://doi.org/10.3390/NU13113951.

24. Bogdan C. Nitric oxide and the immune response. Nat Immunol 2001;2(10): 907–16.

25. Gharavi NM, Baker NA, Mouillesseaux KP, et al. Role of endothelial nitric oxide synthase in the regulation of SREBP activation by oxidized phospholipids. Circ Res 2006;98(6):768–76.

26. Zhivaki D, Kagan JC. Innate immune detection of lipid oxidation as a threat assessment strategy. Nat Rev Immunol 2021. https://doi.org/10.1038/S41577-021-00618-8.

27. Kubes P, Suzuki M, Granger DN. Nitric oxide: an endogenous modulator of leukocyte adhesion. Proc Natl Acad Sci U S A 1991;88(11):4651–5.

28. Kolaczkowska E, Kubes P. Neutrophil recruitment and function in health and inflammation. Nat Rev Immunol 2013;13(3):159–75.

29. Ahluwalia A, Foster P, Scotland RS, et al. Antiinflammatory activity of soluble guanylate cyclase: cGMP-dependent down-regulation of P-selectin expression and leukocyte recruitment. Proc Natl Acad Sci U S A 2004;101(5):1386–91.

30. Geiger R, Rieckmann JC, Wolf T, et al. L-arginine modulates T cell metabolism and enhances survival and anti-tumor activity. Cell 2016;167(3):829–42, e13.

31. Reizine F, Lesouhaitier M, Gregoire M, et al. SARS-CoV-2-induced ARDS associates with MDSC expansion, lymphocyte dysfunction, and arginine shortage. J Clin Immunol 2021;41(3):515–25.
32. Mangoni AA, Rodionov RN, Mcevoy M, et al. New horizons in arginine metabolism, ageing and chronic disease states. Age Ageing 2019;48(6):776–82.
33. Fiorentino G, Coppola A, Izzo R, et al. Effects of adding L-arginine orally to standard therapy in patients with COVID-19: a randomized, double-blind, placebo-controlled, parallel-group trial. Results of the first interim analysis. EClinicalMedicine 2021;40. https://doi.org/10.1016/J.ECLINM.2021.101125.
34. Calvani R, Miccheli A, Landi F, et al. Current nutritional recommendations and novel dietary strategies to manage sarcopenia. J Frailty Aging 2013;2(1):38–53.
35. Piotrowicz K, Gąsowski J, Michel JP, et al. Post-COVID-19 acute sarcopenia: physiopathology and management. Aging Clin Exp Res 2021;33(10):2887–98.
36. Kaczka P, Michalczyk MM, Jastrzab R, et al. Mechanism of action and the effect of beta-hydroxy-beta-methylbutyrate (HMB) supplementation on different types of physical performance - a systematic review. J Hum Kinet 2019;68(1):211–22.
37. Landi F, Calvani R, Picca A, et al. Beta-hydroxy-beta-methylbutyrate and sarcopenia: from biological plausibility to clinical evidence. Curr Opin Clin Nutr Metab Care 2019;22(1):37–43.
38. Bear DE, Langan A, Dimidi E, et al. β-Hydroxy-β-methylbutyrate and its impact on skeletal muscle mass and physical function in clinical practice: a systematic review and meta-analysis. Am J Clin Nutr 2019;109(4):1119–32.
39. Arazi H, Taati B, Suzuki K. A review of the effects of leucine metabolite (β-Hydroxy-β-methylbutyrate) supplementation and resistance training on inflammatory markers: a new approach to oxidative stress and cardiovascular risk factors. Antioxidants (Basel, Switzerland) 2018;7(10). https://doi.org/10.3390/ANTIOX7100148.
40. Hsieh LC, Chien SL, Huang MS, et al. Anti-inflammatory and anticatabolic effects of short-term β-hydroxy-β-methylbutyrate supplementation on chronic obstructive pulmonary disease patients in intensive care unit. Asia Pac J Clin Nutr 2006;15(4):544–50. Available at. https://pubmed.ncbi.nlm.nih.gov/17077073/. Accessed April 13, 2022.
41. Santos-Fandila A, Zafra-Gómez A, Barranco A, et al. Quantitative determination of β-hydroxymethylbutyrate and leucine in culture media and microdialysates from rat brain by UHPLC-tandem mass spectrometry. Anal Bioanal Chem 2014;406(12):2863–72.
42. Salto R, Vílchez JD, Girón MD, et al. β-hydroxy-β-methylbutyrate (HMB) promotes neurite outgrowth in neuro2a cells. PLoS One 2015;10(8). https://doi.org/10.1371/JOURNAL.PONE.0135614.
43. Kougias DG, Nolan SO, Koss WA, et al. Beta-hydroxy-beta-methylbutyrate ameliorates aging effects in the dendritic tree of pyramidal neurons in the medial prefrontal cortex of both male and female rats. Neurobiol Aging 2016;40:78–85.
44. Hankosky ER, Sherrill LK, Ruvola LA, et al. Effects of β-hydroxy-β-methyl butyrate on working memory and cognitive flexibility in an animal model of aging. Nutr Neurosci 2017;20(7):379–87.
45. Kougias DG, Hankosky ER, Gulley JM, et al. Beta-hydroxy-beta-methylbutyrate (HMB) ameliorates age-related deficits in water maze performance, especially in male rats. Physiol Behav 2017;170:93–9.
46. Martínez-Reyes I, Chandel NS. Mitochondrial TCA cycle metabolites control physiology and disease. Nat Commun 2020;11(1). https://doi.org/10.1038/S41467-019-13668-3.

47. Wellen KE, Hatzivassiliou G, Sachdeva UM, et al. ATP-citrate lyase links cellular metabolism to histone acetylation. Science 2009;324(5930):1076–80.
48. Zhang QC, Zhao Y, Bian HM. Anti-thrombotic effect of a novel formula from Corni fructus with malic acid, succinic acid and citric acid. Phytother Res 2014;28(5):722–7.
49. Ruocco C, Segala A, Valerio A, et al. Essential amino acid formulations to prevent mitochondrial dysfunction and oxidative stress. Curr Opin Clin Nutr Metab Care 2021;24(1):88–95.
50. Bifari F, Dolci S, Bottani E, et al. Complete neural stem cell (NSC) neuronal differentiation requires a branched chain amino acids-induced persistent metabolic shift towards energy metabolism. Pharmacol Res 2020;158. https://doi.org/10.1016/J.PHRS.2020.104863.
51. Brunetti D, Bottani E, Segala A, et al. Targeting multiple mitochondrial processes by a metabolic modulator prevents sarcopenia and cognitive decline in SAMP8 mice. Front Pharmacol 2020;11. https://doi.org/10.3389/FPHAR.2020.01171.
52. Bruins MJ, Van Dael P, Eggersdorfer M. The role of nutrients in reducing the risk for noncommunicable diseases during aging. Nutrients 2019;11(1). https://doi.org/10.3390/NU11010085.
53. Calder PC, Carr AC, Gombart AF, et al. Optimal nutritional status for a well-functioning immune system is an important factor to protect against viral infections. Nutrients 2020;12(4). https://doi.org/10.3390/NU12041181.
54. Avery JC, Hoffmann PR. Selenium, selenoproteins, and immunity. Nutrients 2018;10(9). https://doi.org/10.3390/NU10091203.
55. Zhang J, Saad R, Taylor EW, et al. Selenium and selenoproteins in viral infection with potential relevance to COVID-19. Redox Biol 2020;37. https://doi.org/10.1016/j.redox.2020.101715.
56. Bermano G, Meplan C, Mercer DK, et al. Selenium and viral infection: are there lessons for COVID-19? Br J Nutr 2021;125(6):618–27.
57. Hiffler L, Rakotoambinina B. Selenium and RNA virus interactions: potential implications for SARS-CoV-2 infection (COVID-19). Front Nutr 2020;7. https://doi.org/10.3389/FNUT.2020.00164.
58. Kiremidjian-Schumacher L, Roy M, Wishe HI, et al. Supplementation with selenium and human immune cell functions. II. Effect on cytotoxic lymphocytes and natural killer cells. Biol Trace Elem Res 1994;41(1–2):115–27.
59. Giovannini S, Onder G, Lattanzio F, et al. Selenium concentrations and mortality among community-dwelling older adults: results from IISIRENTE study. J Nutr Health Aging 2018;22(5):608–12.
60. Razeghi Jahromi S, Moradi Tabriz H, Togha M, et al. The correlation between serum selenium, zinc, and COVID-19 severity: an observational study. BMC Infect Dis 2021;21(1). https://doi.org/10.1186/S12879-021-06617-3.
61. Dhawan RT, Gopalan D, Howard L, et al. Beyond the clot: perfusion imaging of the pulmonary vasculature after COVID-19. Lancet Respir Med 2021;9(1):107–16.
62. Huang C, Huang L, Wang Y, et al. 6-month consequences of COVID-19 in patients discharged from hospital: a cohort study. Lancet (London, England) 2021;397(10270):220–32.
63. Carfi A, Bernabei R, Landi F. Persistent symptoms in patients after acute COVID-19. JAMA 2020;324(6):603–5.
64. Skalny AV, Timashev PS, Aschner M, et al. Serum zinc, copper, and other biometals are associated with COVID-19 severity markers. Metabolites 2021;11(4). https://doi.org/10.3390/METABO11040244.

65. Majeed M, Nagabhushanam K, Gowda S, et al. An exploratory study of selenium status in healthy individuals and in patients with COVID-19 in a south Indian population: the case for adequate selenium status. Nutrition 2021;82. https://doi.org/10.1016/J.NUT.2020.111053.

66. Bae M, Kim H. Mini-review on the roles of vitamin C, vitamin D, and selenium in the immune system against COVID-19. Molecules 2020;25(22). https://doi.org/10.3390/MOLECULES25225346.

67. Khatiwada S, Subedi A. A mechanistic link between selenium and coronavirus disease 2019 (COVID-19). Curr Nutr Rep 2021;10(2):125–36.

68. Schomburg L. Selenium deficiency due to diet, pregnancy, severe illness, or covid-19-a preventable trigger for autoimmune disease. Int J Mol Sci 2021;22(16). https://doi.org/10.3390/IJMS22168532.

69. Drakesmith H, Prentice A. Viral infection and iron metabolism. Nat Rev Microbiol 2008;6(7):541–52.

70. Liu W, Zhang S, Nekhai S, et al. Depriving iron supply to the virus represents a promising adjuvant therapeutic against viral survival. Curr Clin Microbiol Reports 2020;7(2):13–9.

71. Girelli D, Marchi G, Busti F, et al. Iron metabolism in infections: focus on COVID-19. Semin Hematol 2021;58(3):182–7.

72. Ganz T, Nemeth E. Iron homeostasis in host defence and inflammation. Nat Rev Immunol 2015;15(8):500–10.

73. Shah A, Frost JN, Aaron L, et al. Systemic hypoferremia and severity of hypoxemic respiratory failure in COVID-19. Crit Care 2020;24(1). https://doi.org/10.1186/S13054-020-03051-W.

74. Hippchen T, Altamura S, Muckenthaler MU, et al. Hypoferremia is associated with increased hospitalization and oxygen demand in COVID-19 patients. Hemasphere 2020;4(6). https://doi.org/10.1097/HS9.0000000000000492.

75. Zhao K, Huang J, Dai D, et al. Serum iron level as a potential predictor of coronavirus disease 2019 severity and mortality: a retrospective study. Open Forum Infect Dis 2020;7(7). https://doi.org/10.1093/OFID/OFAA250.

76. Lv Y, Chen L, Liang X, et al. Association between iron status and the risk of adverse outcomes in COVID-19. Clin Nutr 2021;40(5):3462–9.

77. Henry BM, De Oliveira MHS, Benoit S, et al. Hematologic, biochemical and immune biomarker abnormalities associated with severe illness and mortality in coronavirus disease 2019 (COVID-19): a meta-analysis. Clin Chem Lab Med 2020;58(7):1021–8.

78. Cheng L, Li H, Li L, et al. Ferritin in the coronavirus disease 2019 (COVID-19): a systematic review and meta-analysis. J Clin Lab Anal 2020;34(10). https://doi.org/10.1002/JCLA.23618.

79. Huang I, Pranata R, Lim MA, et al. C-reactive protein, procalcitonin, D-dimer, and ferritin in severe coronavirus disease-2019: a meta-analysis. Ther Adv Respir Dis 2020;14. https://doi.org/10.1177/1753466620937175.

80. Sonnweber T, Boehm A, Sahanic S, et al. Persisting alterations of iron homeostasis in COVID-19 are associated with non-resolving lung pathologies and poor patients' performance: a prospective observational cohort study. Respir Res 2020;21(1). https://doi.org/10.1186/S12931-020-01546-2.

81. Pal A, Squitti R, Picozza M, et al. Zinc and COVID-19: basis of current clinical trials. Biol Trace Elem Res 2021;199(8):2882–92.

82. Samad N, Sodunke TE, Abubakar AR, et al. The implications of zinc therapy in combating the COVID-19 global pandemic. J Inflamm Res 2021;14:527–50.

83. Fukada T, Hojyo S, Hara T, et al. Revisiting the old and learning the new of zinc in immunity. Nat Immunol 2019;20(3):248–50.

84. Read SA, Obeid S, Ahlenstiel C, et al. The role of zinc in antiviral immunity. Adv Nutr 2019;10(4):696–710.

85. Skalny AV, Rink L, Ajsuvakova OP, et al. Zinc and respiratory tract infections: perspectives for COVID-19 (review). Int J Mol Med 2020;46(1):17–26.

86. Barnett JB, Hamer DH, Meydani SN. Low zinc status: a new risk factor for pneumonia in the elderly? Nutr Rev 2010;68(1):30–7.

87. Singh M, Das RR. Zinc for the common cold. Cochrane Database Syst Rev 2013;2013(6). https://doi.org/10.1002/14651858.CD001364.PUB4.

88. te Velthuis AJW, van den Worml SHE, Sims AC, et al. Zn(2+) inhibits coronavirus and arterivirus RNA polymerase activity in vitro and zinc ionophores block the replication of these viruses in cell culture. PLoS Pathog 2010;6(11). https://doi.org/10.1371/JOURNAL.PPAT.1001176.

89. Propper RE. Smell/Taste alteration in COVID-19 may reflect zinc deficiency. J Clin Biochem Nutr 2021;68(1):3.

90. Carlucci PM, Ahuja T, Petrilli C, et al. Zinc sulfate in combination with a zinc ionophore may improve outcomes in hospitalized COVID-19 patients. J Med Microbiol 2020;69(10):1228–34.

91. Yao JS, Paguio JA, Dee EC, et al. The Minimal effect of zinc on the survival of hospitalized patients with COVID-19: an observational study. Chest 2021; 159(1):108–11.

92. Thomas S, Patel D, Bittel B, et al. Effect of high-dose zinc and ascorbic acid supplementation vs usual care on symptom length and reduction among ambulatory patients with SARS-CoV-2 infection: the COVID A to Z randomized clinical trial. JAMA Netw Open 2021;4(2). https://doi.org/10.1001/JAMANETWORKOPEN.2021.0369.

93. Wallace TC. Combating COVID-19 and building immune resilience: a potential role for magnesium nutrition? J Am Coll Nutr 2020;39(8):685–93.

94. Tang CF, Ding H, Jiao RQ, et al. Possibility of magnesium supplementation for supportive treatment in patients with COVID-19. Eur J Pharmacol 2020;886. https://doi.org/10.1016/J.EJPHAR.2020.173546.

95. Upala S, Jaruvongvanich V, Wijarnpreecha K, et al. Hypomagnesemia and mortality in patients admitted to intensive care unit: a systematic review and meta-analysis. QJM 2016;109(7):453–9.

96. Iotti S, Wolf F, Mazur A, et al. The COVID-19 pandemic: is there a role for magnesium? Hypotheses and perspectives. Magnes Res 2020;33(2):21–7.

97. Britton J, Pavord I, Richards K, et al. Dietary magnesium, lung function, wheezing, and airway hyperreactivity in a random adult population sample. Lancet 1994;344(8919):357–62.

98. Kew KM, Kirtchuk L, Michell CI. Intravenous magnesium sulfate for treating adults with acute asthma in the emergency department. Cochrane Database Syst Rev 2014;2014(5). https://doi.org/10.1002/14651858.CD010909.

99. Yang Q, Zhang P, Liu T, et al. Magnesium isoglycyrrhizinate ameliorates radiation-induced pulmonary fibrosis by inhibiting fibroblast differentiation via the p38MAPK/Akt/Nox4 pathway. Biomed Pharmacother 2019;115. https://doi.org/10.1016/J.BIOPHA.2019.108955.

100. Chacko SA, Song Y, Nathan L, et al. Relations of dietary magnesium intake to biomarkers of inflammation and endothelial dysfunction in an ethnically diverse cohort of postmenopausal women. Diabetes Care 2010;33(2):304–10.

101. Bermejo-Martin JF, Almansa R, Torres A, et al. COVID-19 as a cardiovascular disease: the potential role of chronic endothelial dysfunction. Cardiovasc Res 2020;116(10):E132–3.

102. Darooghegi Mofrad M, Djafarian K, Mozaffari H, et al. Effect of magnesium supplementation on endothelial function: a systematic review and meta-analysis of randomized controlled trials. Atherosclerosis 2018;273:98–105.

103. Tan CW, Ho LP, Kalimuddin S, et al. Cohort study to evaluate the effect of vitamin D, magnesium, and vitamin B 12 in combination on progression to severe outcomes in older patients with coronavirus (COVID-19). Nutrition 2020;79–80.

104. Chakraborty AJ, Mitra S, Tallei TE, et al. Bromelain a potential bioactive compound: a comprehensive overview from a pharmacological perspective. Life (Basel) 2021;11(4). https://doi.org/10.3390/LIFE11040317.

105. Bhui K, Prasad S, George J, et al. Bromelain inhibits COX-2 expression by blocking the activation of MAPK regulated NF-kappa B against skin tumor-initiation triggering mitochondrial death pathway. Cancer Lett 2009;282(2): 167–76.

106. Taussig SJ, Batkin S. Bromelain, the enzyme complex of pineapple (Ananas comosus) and its clinical application. An update. J Ethnopharmacol 1988;22(2): 191–203.

107. Metzig C, Grabowska E, Eckert K, et al. Bromelain proteases reduce human platelet aggregation in vitro, adhesion to bovine endothelial cells and thrombus formation in rat vessels in Vivo. In Vivo (Brooklyn) 1999;13(1):7–12.

108. Kumakura S, Yamashita M, Tsurufuji S. Effect of bromelain on kaolin-induced inflammation in rats. Eur J Pharmacol 1988;150(3):295–301.

109. Engwerda CR, Andrew D, Ladhams A, et al. Bromelain modulates T cell and B cell immune responses in vitro and in vivo. Cell Immunol 2001;210(1):66–75.

110. Sagar S, Rathinavel AK, Lutz WE, et al. Bromelain inhibits SARS-CoV-2 infection via targeting ACE-2, TMPRSS2, and spike protein. Clin Transl Med 2021;11(2). https://doi.org/10.1002/CTM2.281.

111. Kritis P, Karampela I, Kokoris S, et al. The combination of bromelain and curcumin as an immune-boosting nutraceutical in the prevention of severe COVID-19. Metab Open 2020;8:100066.

112. Zamanian M, Bazmandegan G, Sureda A, et al. The protective roles and molecular mechanisms of troxerutin (vitamin p4) for the treatment of chronic diseases: a mechanistic review. Curr Neuropharmacol 2021;19(1):97–110.

113. Panat NA, Maurya DK, Ghaskadbi SS, et al. Troxerutin, a plant flavonoid, protects cells against oxidative stress-induced cell death through radical scavenging mechanism. Food Chem 2016;194:32–45.

114. Farajdokht F, Amani M, Bavil FM, et al. Troxerutin protects hippocampal neurons against amyloid beta-induced oxidative stress and apoptosis. EXCLI J 2017;16: 1081–9.

115. Salama SA, Arab HH, Maghrabi IA. Troxerutin down-regulates KIM-1, modulates p38 MAPK signaling, and enhances renal regenerative capacity in a rat model of gentamycin-induced acute kidney injury. Food Funct 2018; 9(12):6632–42.

116. Ahmadi Z, Mohammadinejad R, Roomiani S, et al. Biological and therapeutic effects of troxerutin: molecular signaling pathways come into view. J Pharmacopuncture 2021;24(1):1–13.

117. Azarfarin M, Farajdokht F, Babri S, et al. Effects of troxerutin on anxiety- and depressive-like behaviors induced by chronic mild stress in adult male rats. Iran J Basic Med Sci 2018;21(8):781–6.

118. Zavvari Oskuye Z, Mirzaei Bavil F, Hamidian GHR, et al. Troxerutin affects the male fertility in prepubertal type 1 diabetic male rats. Iran J Basic Med Sci 2019;22(2):197–205.

119. Yu Y, Zheng G. Troxerutin protects against diabetic cardiomyopathy through NF-κB/AKT/IRS1 in a rat model of type 2 diabetes. Mol Med Rep 2017;15(6): 3473–8.

120. Siqueiros-Cendón T, Arévalo-Gallegos S, Iglesias-Figueroa BF, et al. Immuno-modulatory effects of lactoferrin. Acta Pharmacol Sin 2014;35(5):557–66.

121. Bruni N, Capucchio MT, Biasibetti E, et al. Antimicrobial activity of lactoferrin-related peptides and applications in human and veterinary medicine. Molecules 2016;21(6). https://doi.org/10.3390/MOLECULES21060752.

122. Valenti P, Antonini G. Lactoferrin: an important host defence against microbial and viral attack. Cell Mol Life Sci 2005;62(22):2576–87.

123. Pietrantoni A, Dofrelli E, Tinari A, et al. Bovine lactoferrin inhibits influenza A virus induced programmed cell death in vitro. Biometals 2010;23(3):465–75.

124. Beljaars L, Van Der Strate BWA, Bakker HI, et al. Inhibition of cytomegalovirus infection by lactoferrin in vitro and in vivo. Antivir Res 2004;63(3):197–208.

125. Andersen JH, Jenssen H, Sandvik K, et al. Anti-HSV activity of lactoferrin and lactoferricin is dependent on the presence of heparan sulphate at the cell surface. J Med Virol 2004;74(2):262–71.

126. Berlutti F, Pantanella F, Natalizi T, et al. Antiviral properties of lactoferrin–a natural immunity molecule. Molecules 2011;16(8):6992–7012.

127. Chang R, Ng TB, Sun WZ. Lactoferrin as potential preventative and adjunct treatment for COVID-19. Int J Antimicrob Agents 2020;56(3). https://doi.org/10.1016/J.IJANTIMICAG.2020.106118.

128. Campione E, Lanna C, Cosio T, et al. Lactoferrin against SARS-CoV-2: in vitro and in silico evidences. Front Pharmacol 2021;12. https://doi.org/10.3389/FPHAR.2021.666600.

129. Rosa L, Cutone A, Lepanto MS, et al. Lactoferrin: a natural glycoprotein involved in iron and inflammatory homeostasis. Int J Mol Sci 2017;18(9). https://doi.org/10.3390/IJMS18091985.

130. Campione E, Lanna C, Cosio T, et al. Lactoferrin as antiviral treatment in COVID-19 management: preliminary evidence. Int J Environ Res Public Health 2021; 18(20). https://doi.org/10.3390/IJERPH182010985.

131. Zhong P, Xu J, Yang D, et al. COVID-19-associated gastrointestinal and liver injury: clinical features and potential mechanisms. Signal Transduct Target Ther 2020;5(1). https://doi.org/10.1038/S41392-020-00373-7.

132. Wu Y, Guo C, Tang L, et al. Prolonged presence of SARS-CoV-2 viral RNA in faecal samples. Lancet Gastroenterol Hepatol 2020;5(5):434–5.

133. Yeoh YK, Zuo T, Lui GCY, et al. Gut microbiota composition reflects disease severity and dysfunctional immune responses in patients with COVID-19. Gut 2021;70(4):698–706.

134. Hussain I, Cher GLY, Abid MA, et al. Role of gut microbiome in COVID-19: an insight into pathogenesis and therapeutic potential. Front Immunol 2021;12. https://doi.org/10.3389/FIMMU.2021.765965.

135. Liu Q, Mak JWY, Su Q, et al. Gut microbiota dynamics in a prospective cohort of patients with post-acute COVID-19 syndrome. Gut 2022;71(3):544–52.

136. Hill C, Guarner F, Reid G, et al. Expert consensus document. the international scientific association for probiotics and Prebiotics consensus statement on the scope and appropriate use of the term probiotic. Nat Rev Gastroenterol Hepatol 2014;11(8):506–14.

137. Dang AT, Marsland BJ. Microbes, metabolites, and the gut-lung axis. Mucosal Immunol 2019;12(4):843–50.

138. Yahfoufi N, Mallet JF, Graham E, et al. Role of probiotics and prebiotics in immunomodulation. Curr Opin Food Sci 2018;20:82–91.

139. Cristofori F, Dargenio VN, Dargenio C, et al. Anti-inflammatory and immunomodulatory effects of probiotics in gut inflammation: a door to the body. Front Immunol 2021;12. https://doi.org/10.3389/FIMMU.2021.578386.

140. Wang Y, Wu Y, Wang Y, et al. Antioxidant properties of probiotic bacteria. Nutrients 2017;9(5). https://doi.org/10.3390/NU9050521.

141. Mirashrafi S, Moravejolahkami AR, Balouch Zehi Z, et al. The efficacy of probiotics on virus titres and antibody production in virus diseases: a systematic review on recent evidence for COVID-19 treatment. Clin Nutr ESPEN 2021;46:1–8. https://doi.org/10.1016/J.CLNESP.2021.10.016.

142. Rather IA, Choi SB, Kamli MR, et al. Potential adjuvant therapeutic effect of lactobacillus plantarum probio-88 postbiotics against SARS-COV-2. Vaccines 2021;9(10). https://doi.org/10.3390/VACCINES9101067.

143. Salaris C, Scarpa M, Elli M, et al. Lacticaseibacillus paracasei DG enhances the lactoferrin anti-SARS-CoV-2 response in Caco-2 cells. Gut Microbes 2021;13(1). https://doi.org/10.1080/19490976.2021.1961970.

144. Nguyen QV, Chong LC, Hor YY, et al. Role of probiotics in the management of COVID-19: a computational perspective. Nutrients 2022;14(2). https://doi.org/10.3390/NU14020274.

145. d'Ettorre G, Ceccarelli G, Marazzato M, et al. Challenges in the management of SARS-CoV2 infection: the role of oral bacteriotherapy as complementary therapeutic strategy to avoid the progression of COVID-19. Front Med 2020;7. https://doi.org/10.3389/FMED.2020.00389.

146. Li Q, Cheng F, Xu Q, et al. The role of probiotics in coronavirus disease-19 infection in Wuhan: a retrospective study of 311 severe patients. Int Immunopharmacol 2021;95. https://doi.org/10.1016/J.INTIMP.2021.107531.

147. Gutiérrez-Castrellón P, Gandara-Martí T, Abreu Y Abreu AT, et al. Probiotic improves symptomatic and viral clearance in Covid19 outpatients: a randomized, quadruple-blinded, placebo-controlled trial. Gut Microbes 2022;14(1). https://doi.org/10.1080/19490976.2021.2018899.

148. Bouillon R, Marcocci C, Carmeliet G, et al. Skeletal and extraskeletal actions of vitamin D: current evidence and outstanding questions. Endocr Rev 2019;40(4):1109–51.

149. Charoenngam N, Holick MF. Immunologic effects of vitamin D on human health and disease. Nutrients 2020;12(7):1–28.

150. Gombart AF. The vitamin D-antimicrobial peptide pathway and its role in protection against infection. Future Microbiol 2009;4(9):1151–65.

151. Rak K, Bronkowska M. Immunomodulatory effect of vitamin D and its potential role in the prevention and treatment of type 1 diabetes mellitus-a narrative review. Molecules 2018;24(1). https://doi.org/10.3390/MOLECULES24010053.

152. Littorin B, Blom P, Schölin A, et al. Lower levels of plasma 25-hydroxyvitamin D among young adults at diagnosis of autoimmune type 1 diabetes compared with control subjects: results from the nationwide diabetes incidence study in Sweden (DISS). Diabetologia 2006;49(12):2847–52.

153. Mokry LE, Ross S, Ahmad OS, et al. Vitamin D and risk of multiple sclerosis: a mendelian randomization study. Plos Med 2015;12(8). https://doi.org/10.1371/JOURNAL.PMED.1001866.
154. Sainaghi PP, Bellan M, Carda S, et al. Hypovitaminosis D and response to cholecalciferol supplementation in patients with autoimmune and non-autoimmune rheumatic diseases. Rheumatol Int 2012;32(11):3365–72.
155. Monlezun DJ, Bittner EA, Christopher KB, et al. Vitamin D status and acute respiratory infection: cross sectional results from the United States national health and nutrition examination survey, 2001-2006. Nutrients 2015;7(3):1933–44.
156. Baktash V, Hosack T, Patel N, et al. Vitamin D status and outcomes for hospitalised older patients with COVID-19. Postgrad Med J 2021;97(1149):442–7.
157. Chiodini I, Gatti D, Soranna D, et al. Vitamin D status and SARS-CoV-2 infection and COVID-19 clinical outcomes. Front Public Heal 2021;9. https://doi.org/10.3389/FPUBH.2021.736665.
158. Rastogi A, Bhansali A, Khare N, et al. Short term, high-dose vitamin D supplementation for COVID-19 disease: a randomised, placebo-controlled, study (SHADE study). Postgrad Med J 2022;98(1156):87–90.
159. Annweiler C, Beaudenon M, Simon R, et al. Vitamin D supplementation prior to or during COVID-19 associated with better 3-month survival in geriatric patients: extension phase of the GERIA-COVID study. J Steroid Biochem Mol Biol 2021; 213. https://doi.org/10.1016/J.JSBMB.2021.105958.
160. Stroehlein JK, Wallqvist J, Iannizzi C, et al. Vitamin D supplementation for the treatment of COVID-19: a living systematic review. Cochrane Database Syst Rev 2021;5(5). https://doi.org/10.1002/14651858.CD015043.
161. Townsend L, Dyer AH, McCluskey P, et al. Investigating the relationship between vitamin D and persistent symptoms following SARS-CoV-2 infection. Nutrients 2021;13(7). https://doi.org/10.3390/NU13072430.
162. Remelli F, Vitali A, Zurlo A, et al. Vitamin D deficiency and sarcopenia in older persons. Nutrients 2019;11(12). https://doi.org/10.3390/NU11122861.
163. Genazzani A, Panay N, Simoncini T, et al. Purified and specific cytoplasmic pollen extract: a non-hormonal alternative for the treatment of menopausal symptoms. Gynecol Endocrinol 2020;36(3):190–6.
164. Komosinska-Vassev K, Olczyk P, Kaźmierczak J, et al. Bee pollen: chemical composition and therapeutic application. Evid Based Complement Alternat Med 2015;2015. https://doi.org/10.1155/2015/297425.
165. LELLO S, CAPOZZI A, XHOLLI A, et al. The benefits of purified cytoplasm of pollen in reducing menopausal symptoms in peri- and post-menopause: an Italian multicentre prospective observational study. *Minerva Obstet Gynecol* November 2021. https://doi.org/10.23736/S2724-606X.21.04964-2.
166. Hellström AC, Muntzing J. The pollen extract Femal–a nonestrogenic alternative to hormone therapy in women with menopausal symptoms. Menopause 2012; 19(7):825–9.
167. Fait T, Sailer M, Regidor PA. Prospective observational study to evaluate the efficacy and safety of the pollen extract Sérélys ® in the management of women with menopausal symptoms. Gynecol Endocrinol 2019;35(4):360–3.
168. Mirmiran P, Houshialsadat Z, Gaeini Z, et al. Functional properties of beetroot (Beta vulgaris) in management of cardio-metabolic diseases. Nutr Metab (Lond) 2020;17(1). https://doi.org/10.1186/S12986-019-0421-0.
169. Milton-Laskibar I, Alfredo Martínez J, Portillo MP. Current knowledge on beetroot bioactive compounds: role of nitrate and betalains in health and disease. Foods (Basel, Switzerland) 2021;10(6). https://doi.org/10.3390/FOODS10061314.

170. Lundberg JO, Weitzberg E, Gladwin MT. The nitrate-nitrite-nitric oxide pathway in physiology and therapeutics. Nat Rev Drug Discov 2008;7(2):156–67.
171. Kapil V, Khambata RS, Jones DA, et al. The noncanonical pathway for in vivo nitric oxide generation: the nitrate-nitrite-nitric oxide pathway. Pharmacol Rev 2020;72(3):692–766.
172. Jones AM, Thompson C, Wylie LJ, et al. Dietary nitrate and physical performance. Annu Rev Nutr 2018;38:303–28.
173. Larsen FJ, Weitzberg E, Lundberg JO, et al. Effects of dietary nitrate on oxygen cost during exercise. Acta Physiol (Oxf) 2007;191(1):59–66.
174. Arazi H, Eghbali E. Possible effects of beetroot supplementation on physical performance through metabolic, neuroendocrine, and antioxidant mechanisms: a narrative review of the literature. Front Nutr 2021;8. https://doi.org/10.3389/FNUT.2021.660150.
175. Walker MA, Bailey TG, McIlvenna L, et al. Acute dietary nitrate supplementation improves flow mediated dilatation of the superficial femoral artery in healthy older males. Nutrients 2019;11(5). https://doi.org/10.3390/NU11050954.
176. Pekas EJ, Wooden TSK, Yadav SK, et al. Body mass-normalized moderate dose of dietary nitrate intake improves endothelial function and walking capacity in patients with peripheral artery disease. Am J Physiol Regul Integr Comp Physiol 2021;321(2):R162–73.
177. Volino-Souza M, De Oliveira GV, Alvares TS. A single dose of beetroot juice improves endothelial function but not tissue oxygenation in pregnant women: a randomised clinical trial. Br J Nutr 2018;120(9):1006–13.
178. Velmurugan S, Gan JM, Rathod KS, et al. Dietary nitrate improves vascular function in patients with hypercholesterolemia: a randomized, double-blind, placebo-controlled study. Am J Clin Nutr 2016;103(1):25–38.
179. Kapil V, Khambata RS, Robertson A, et al. Dietary nitrate provides sustained blood pressure lowering in hypertensive patients: a randomized, phase 2, double-blind, placebo-controlled study. Hypertens 2015;65(2):320–7.
180. Vanhatalo A, Bailey SJ, Blackwell JR, et al. Acute and chronic effects of dietary nitrate supplementation on blood pressure and the physiological responses to moderate-intensity and incremental exercise. Am J Physiol Regul Integr Comp Physiol 2010;299(4).
181. Asgary S, Afshani MR, Sahebkar A, et al. Improvement of hypertension, endothelial function and systemic inflammation following short-term supplementation with red beet (Beta vulgaris L.) juice: a randomized crossover pilot study. J Hum Hypertens 2016;30(10):627–32.
182. Kelly J, Fulford J, Vanhatalo A, et al. Effects of short-term dietary nitrate supplementation on blood pressure, O2 uptake kinetics, and muscle and cognitive function in older adults. Am J Physiol Regul Integr Comp Physiol 2013;304(2). https://doi.org/10.1152/AJPREGU.00406.2012.
183. Ocampo DAB, Paipilla AF, Marín E, et al. Dietary nitrate from beetroot juice for hypertension: a systematic review. Biomolecules 2018;8(4). https://doi.org/10.3390/BIOM8040134.
184. Kroll JL, Werchan CA, Rosenfield D, et al. Acute ingestion of beetroot juice increases exhaled nitric oxide in healthy individuals. PLoS One 2018;13(1). https://doi.org/10.1371/JOURNAL.PONE.0191030.
185. Alshafie S, El-Helw GO, Fayoud AM, et al. Efficacy of dietary nitrate-rich beetroot juice supplementation in patients with chronic obstructive pulmonary disease (COPD): a systematic review and meta-analysis. Clin Nutr ESPEN 2021;42:32–40.

186. Raubenheimer K, Hickey D, Leveritt M, et al. Acute effects of nitrate-rich beetroot juice on blood pressure, hemostasis and vascular inflammation markers in healthy older adults: a randomized, placebo-controlled crossover study. Nutrients 2017;9(11).

187. Clifford T, Howatson G, West DJ, et al. The potential benefits of red beetroot supplementation in health and disease. Nutrients 2015;7(4):2801–22.

188. Polturak G, Aharoni A. La Vie en Rose": biosynthesis, sources, and applications of betalain pigments. Mol Plant 2018;11(1):7–22.

189. Kanner J, Harel S, Granit R. Betalains–a new class of dietary cationized antioxidants. J Agric Food Chem 2001;49(11):5178–85.

190. Krajka-Kuźniak V, Paluszczak J, Szaefer H, et al. Betanin, a beetroot component, induces nuclear factor erythroid-2-related factor 2-mediated expression of detoxifying/antioxidant enzymes in human liver cell lines. Br J Nutr 2013; 110(12):2138–49.

191. Reddy MK, Alexander-Lindo RL, Nair MG. Relative inhibition of lipid peroxidation, cyclooxygenase enzymes, and human tumor cell proliferation by natural food colors. J Agric Food Chem 2005;53(23):9268–73.

192. Vidal PJ, López-Nicolás JM, Gandía-Herrero F, et al. Inactivation of lipoxygenase and cyclooxygenase by natural betalains and semi-synthetic analogues. Food Chem 2014;154:246–54.

193. Silva DVT da, Baião D dos S, Ferreira VF, et al. Betanin as a multipath oxidative stress and inflammation modulator: a beetroot pigment with protective effects on cardiovascular disease pathogenesis. Crit Rev Food Sci Nutr 2022;62(2): 539–54.

194. Moreno-Ley CM, Osorio-Revilla G, Hernández-Martínez DM, et al. Anti-inflammatory activity of betalains: a comprehensive review. Hum Nutr Metab 2021; 25:200126.

195. Pietrzkowski Z, Nemzer B, Sporna A, et al. Influence of betalain-rich extract on reduction of discomfort associated with osteoarthritisa) • New Medicine 1/2010. Czytelnia Medyczna Borgis 2009;(1). Available at. http://www. czytelniamedyczna.pl/3333,influence-of-betalainrich-extract-on-reduction-of-discomfort-associated-with-ost.html. Accessed April 13, 2022.

196. Volino-Souza M, Oliveira GV de, Conte-Junior CA, et al. Covid-19 quarantine: impact of lifestyle behaviors changes on endothelial function and possible protective effect of beetroot juice. Front Nutr 2020;7. https://doi.org/10.3389/FNUT. 2020.582210.

197. Giampaoli O, Sciubba F, Conta G, et al. Red Beetroot's NMR-based metabolomics: phytochemical profile related to development time and production year. Foods (Basel, Switzerland) 2021;10(8). https://doi.org/10.3390/FOODS10081887.

198. Landi F, Cesari M, Calvani R, et al. The "Sarcopenia and Physical fRailty IN older people: multi-componenT Treatment strategies" (SPRINTT) randomized controlled trial: design and methods. Aging Clin Exp Res 2017;29(1): 89–100.

199. Salini S, Russo A, Biscotti D, et al. Professional sport players recover from coronavirus and return to competition: hopes for resuming a normal life after COVID-19 for older people. J Gerontol Geriatr 2020;68(Special issue 4): 212–5.

200. Hashimoto S, Yoshizaki K, Uno K, et al. Prompt Reduction in CRP, IL-6, IFN-γ, IP-10, and MCP-1 and a Relatively Low Basal Ratio of Ferritin/CRP Is Possibly Associated With the Efficacy of Tocilizumab Monotherapy in Severely to

Critically Ill Patients With COVID-19. Front Med (Lausanne) 2021;8:734838. https://doi.org/10.3389/fmed.2021.734838. Published 2021 Sep 23.

FURTHER READING

Hashimoto Shoji, Yoshizaki Kazuyuki, Uno Kazuko, et al. Prompt Reduction in CRP, IL-6, IFN-γ, IP-10, and MCP-1 and a Relatively Low Basal Ratio of Ferritin/CRP Is Possibly Associated With the Efficacy of Tocilizumab Monotherapy in Severely to Critically Ill Patients With COVID-19. Frontiers in medicine 2021;8. https://doi.org/10.3389/fmed.2021.734838.

Neuropsychological Measures of Long COVID-19 Fog in Older Subjects

Alessandra Lauria, MD, Angelo Carfì, MD*,
Francesca Benvenuto, MD, Giulia Bramato, MD,
Francesca Ciciarello, MD, Sara Rocchi, MD, Elisabetta Rota, MD,
Andrea Salerno, MD, Leonardo Stella, MD, Marcello Tritto, MD,
Antonella Di Paola, Psy.D, Cristina Pais, MD, Matteo Tosato, MD,
Delfina Janiri, MD, Gabriele Sani, MD,
Francesco Cosimo Pagano, MD, Massimo Fantoni, MD,
Roberto Bernabei, MD, Francesco Landi, MD,
Alessandra Bizzarro, MD, on behalf of Gemelli Against COVID-19
Post-acute Care Study Group[1]

KEYWORDS

- Long COVID • Elderly • Cognitive impairment

KEY POINTS

- We asked whether coronavirus disease 2019 can have a long-term impact on cognitive function in the elderly.
- In this cohort study of 100 elderly individuals assessed on average 3 months after acute coronavirus disease 2019, we found a high prevalence of failed neuropsychological tests.
- We found that coronavirus disease 2019 is capable of eliciting persistent measurable neurocognitive alterations in the elderly, particularly in the areas of attention and working memory.

INTRODUCTION

Since December 2019, when the first cases of the coronavirus disease 2019 (COVID-19) were confirmed in the Chinese Hubei region, the pandemic of severe acute

The authors declare to have no conflicts of interest.
Funded by: ITALYLETR.
Gemelli Against COVID-19 Post-acute Care Study Group, Fondazione Policlinico Universitario Agostino Gemelli IRCCS, Largo F. Vito 1, Rome 00168, Italy
[1] The full list of authors in the study group is uploaded in the Resources/Supplementary file.
* Corresponding author. Centro Medicina dell'Invecchiamento, Fondazione Policlinico Universitario "A. Gemelli" IRCCS, Largo F. Vito 1, Rome 00168, Italy.
E-mail address: angelo.carfi@policlinicogemelli.it

respiratory syndrome coronavirus 2 continues to plague populations and health systems around the world. A number of descriptions now cover the long-term symptoms of the disease, which include fatigue, shortness of breath, and pain.[1,2] Neurologic involvement and psychological symptoms owing to or related to the disease are described to affect up to one-third of infected people.[3–5] These symptoms include a wide spectrum of manifestations that are often loosely described as a general mental slowness often named foggy brain or COVID fog.[6] Such symptoms can characterize both the acute phase and the convalescent period, during which patients report an ill-defined sense of not feeling their best or of not having fully recovered their previous well-being in the physical, occupational, or social domains.[7] In some studies, cognitive problems were tied to a diagnosis of dementia[5] and concern is particularly high for the aged populations.

Because the availability of clinical data remains poor, the aim of the present study was to investigate the neurologic and cognitive features of a sample of elderly patients with confirmed diagnosis of COVID-19 evaluated in the postacute phase through a direct neuropsychological evaluation.

METHODS

Since April 21, 2020, a postacute outpatient service for individuals recovering from COVID-19 was established at our institution. All patients with a previous diagnosis of COVID-19 who met criteria for discontinuation of quarantine were considered eligible (no fever for 3 consecutive days, improvement in other symptoms, and 2 negative test results for severe acute respiratory syndrome coronavirus 2 taken 24 hours apart).

Once enrolled, each participant underwent a number of evaluations (described elsewere[8]), including a detailed history, neurologic objective examination, and specific anamnesis for general and neurologic symptomatology. For the purpose of this study, we enrolled individuals over the age of 65 years.

Cognitive Evaluation

After the anamnestic evaluation and neurologic objectivity, each patient underwent a neuropsychological evaluation that included Mini Mental State Examination[9] and 8 more specific neuropsychological tests: the Rey Auditory Verbal Test was used to investigate immediate and deferred memory[10]; selective attention and visual–spatial exploration were assessed with Multiple Features Target Cancellation Test[11,12]; the Trial Making Test assessed selective, divided, and alternating, attention together with other features such as psychomotor speed, visuospatial research ability and working memory[13,14]; the Digit Span Forward and Backward evaluated the verbal short-term and working memory capacity[15]; and the Frontal Assessment Battery evaluates composite multidimensional domains and was used to screen for global executive dysfunction including behavioral, affective, motivational and cognitive components.[16,17]

Of each neuropsychological test were reported the raw scores, the scores adjusted for age and educational level and gender (where appropriate), and standardized scores on a 5-point ordinal scale (Equivalent Scores).[18] A test Equivalent Score of 0 was considered pathologic, a score of 1 was classified as borderline, and scores of 2 to 5 were considered consistent with normal performance.

Other Evaluations

Psychiatric domains were evaluated with the Hamilton Anxiety[19,20] and Depression[21,22] scales and the Kessler Psychological Distress scales,[23,24] and anxiety, depressive symptoms, and global psychological distress were evaluated with a cut-off of 7, 7, and 19 in each scale total score, respectively. The Pittsburg Sleep Quality Index[25] was used to assess sleep quality and disturbances.

Case severity was assessed with the 7-category ordinal scale,[26] which classifies participants based on the need for hospitalization and O_2 administration into 1 to 2, nonhospitalized; 3, hospitalized, not requiring supplemental oxygen; 4, hospitalized, requiring supplemental oxygen; 5, hospitalized, requiring nasal high-flow oxygen therapy, noninvasive mechanical ventilation, or both; 6, hospitalized, requiring invasive mechanical ventilation, extracorporeal membrane oxygenation, or both; and 7, death. Given the differences in the clinical manifestations and severity between sexes,[27] results were also compared by sex.

Statistical Analysis

Descriptive analyses and comparisons were obtained through ANOVA and χ^2 tests where appropriate. The P value was set to less than .05 for statistical significance. Given the descriptive basis of the analyses no correction of significance levels was used. All analyses were conducted using R version 4.1.3 (R Foundation, Vienna, Austria).

This study was approved by the Università Cattolica and Fondazione Policlinico Gemelli IRCCS Institutional Ethics Committee. Written informed consent was obtained from all participants.

RESULTS

We present data from 100 individuals (mean age, 73.4 ± 6.1 years; 35% female) assessed at our institution from April 23, 2020, to November 30, 2020. The general characteristics of the study participants, stratified by sex, are described in **Table 1**. Females presented a lower prevalence of diabetes mellitus and a higher prevalence of thyroid disorders. In contrast, males showed less persistence of post–COVID-19 symptoms and on average a smaller decrease in quality-of-life scores.

On average, the assessment was performed 96.5 days after the onset of COVID-19 symptoms. Fatigue was reported by half of the enrolled participants; apart from that, as shown in **Fig. 1**, very high rates of persistent neurologic symptoms were reported in the domains of memory, attention, and sleep. The outcome of neuropsychological testing is described in **Table 2** and **Fig. 2**. On average, the adjusted Mini Mental State Exam score was 28.2 ± 1.7, as expected in a study sample consisting of fairly educated individuals with no history of cognitive impairment. No significant differences were observed within the severity groups. Importantly, 33%, 23%, and 20% of participants achieved either pathologic or borderline performances on the Trial Making, Digit Span Backwards, and Frontal Evaluation Battery tests, respectively. It is also notable that on the neuropsychological assessment a total of 33 participants were found to perform at a level considered to be pathologic.

DISCUSSION

This single-center study investigated the cognitive status of a group of elderly people post–COVID-19 through a battery of neuropsychological tests. Interviewed on average 3 months after the onset of the first symptoms of COVID-19, a significant

Table 1
Sample characteristics

	Total n = 100	Males n = 65	Females n = 35	p
General information				
Age (years)	73.4 (6.1)	73.4 (5.8)	73.5 (6.7)	0.957
Females	35 (35%)			
BMI (kg/m^2)	26.1 (3.9)	26.2 (3.7)	25.9 (4.1)	0.695
Education (years)	12.7 (8.7)	13.0 (5.5)	12.2 (12.7)	0.678
Not employed	80 (80%)	51 (78.5%)	29 (82.9%)	0.793
Flu vaccination	53 (53%)	40 (61.5%)	13 (37.1%)	0.046
Antipneumococcal vaccination	21 (21%)	17 (26.2%)	4 (11.4%)	0.16
Regular physical activity	60 (60%)	37 (56.9%)	23 (65.7%)	0.784
Smoking status				0.115
Nonsmoker	37 (37%)	20 (30.8%)	17 (48.6%)	
Active smoker	6 (6%)	5 (7.7%)	1 (2.9%)	
Former smoker	52 (52%)	38 (58.5%)	14 (40%)	
Unknown	5 (5%)	2 (3.1%)	3 (8.6%)	
Pre-COVID clinical features				
Cardiovascular conditions	69 (69%)	49 (75.4%)	20 (57.1%)	0.098
Chronic heart disease	19 (19%)	16 (24.6%)	3 (8.6%)	0.092
Atrial fibrillation	12 (12%)	7 (10.8%)	5 (14.3%)	0.847
Heart failure	8 (8%)	6 (9.2%)	2 (5.7%)	0.817
Stroke	2 (2%)	0 (0%)	2 (5.7%)	0.231
Hypertension	58 (58%)	41 (63.1%)	17 (48.6%)	0.234
Diabetes mellitus	19 (19%)	17 (26.2%)	2 (5.7%)	0.027
Renal failure	9 (9%)	6 (9.2%)	3 (8.6%)	1
Thyroid disease	24 (24%)	9 (13.8%)	15 (42.9%)	0.003
COPD	22 (22%)	15 (23.1%)	7 (20%)	0.919
Active cancer	7 (7%)	4 (6.2%)	3 (8.6%)	0.967
Immune disease	8 (8%)	3 (4.6%)	5 (14.3%)	0.189
COVID-19 events				
Seven category ordinal scale				0.092
2. Not hospitalized	12 (12%)	5 (7.7%)	7 (20%)	
3. Hospitalized, not requiring O$_2$	14 (14%)	6 (9.2%)	8 (22.9%)	
4. Hospitalized, requiring O$_2$	43 (43%)	31 (47.7%)	12 (34.3%)	
5. Hospitalized, requiring HFNC/NIV	16 (16%)	12 (18.5%)	4 (11.4%)	
6. Hospitalized, requiring intubation/ECMO	15 (15%)	11 (16.9%)	4 (11.4%)	
Drug treatments				
Treatment for COVID-19 pneumonia	81 (81%)	56 (86.2%)	25 (71.4%)	0.128
Anti retrovirals	80 (80%)	56 (86.2%)	24 (68.6%)	0.067
Hydroxychloroquine	80 (80%)	55 (84.6%)	25 (71.4%)	0.19
Anti-IL6	40 (40%)	29 (44.6%)	11 (31.4%)	0.29
Azithromycin	42 (42%)	31 (47.7%)	11 (31.4%)	0.174
Other antibiotics	48 (48%)	35 (53.8%)	13 (37.1%)	0.166

(continued on next page)

Table 1
(continued)

	Total	Males	Females	p
	n = 100	n = 65	n = 35	
Enoxaparin	73 (73%)	47 (72.3%)	26 (74.3%)	1
Corticosteroids	15 (15%)	9 (13.8%)	6 (17.1%)	0.883
Antiplatelet drugs	19 (19%)	16 (24.6%)	3 (8.6%)	0.092
Length of stay (days)	23.3 (16.1)	25.4 (15.8)	18.8 (16.0)	0.072
Post COVID-19				
Days since first symptoms	96.5 (45.3)	93.2 (40.7)	102.7 (52.8)	0.319
Days since hospital discharge	62.1 (39.7)	58.3 (34.4)	70.2 (48.9)	0.25
N. persistent symptoms	3.0 (2.5)	2.6 (2.3)	3.8 (2.9)	0.02
Persistent symptoms				0.114
No symptoms	17 (17%)	14 (21.5%)	3 (8.6%)	
1–2 symptoms	33 (33%)	23 (35.4%)	10 (28.6%)	
≥3 symptoms	50 (50%)	28 (43.1%)	22 (62.9%)	
Decrease in QoL (EQ-VAS)	−10.1 (14.0)	−7.7 (13.1)	−14.7 (14.8)	0.022

Abbreviations: BMI, body mass index; COPD, chronic obstructive pulmonary disease; ECMO, extra-corporeal membrane oxygenation; EQ-VAS, EuroQol visual analog scale; HFNC, high-flow nasal cannulae; NIV, noninvasive ventilation; QoL, quality of life.

proportion of participants reported persistent sleep (33%), attention (30%), and memory (30%) symptoms. These findings are consistent with several previous studies[5,28] and the well-established notion that COVID-19 leaves behind a burden of persistent symptoms pertaining to many organ systems.[1]

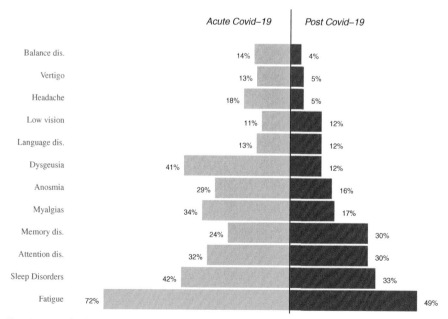

Fig. 1. Neurologic symptoms reported in the acute and recovery phase.

Table 2
Neuropsychological tests

	Total	Sex				Severity – Seven Category Ordinal Scale					
						Not Hospitalized	Hospitalized				
		Males	Females	P Value		2. At Home	3. No O$_2$	4. O$_2$	5. HFNC/NIV	6. Intubation/ECMO	P Value
	n = 100	n = 65	n = 35			n = 12	n = 14	n = 43	n = 16	n = 15	
MMSE											
Corrected	28.2 (1.7)	28.4 (1.7)	27.7 (1.8)	0.068		28.2 (1.9)	28.5 (1.5)	27.9 (2.1)	28.2 (1.3)	28.7 (0.8)	0.48
Rey's immediate recall											
Corrected	42.6 (7.8)	41.8 (8.0)	44.1 (7.3)	0.171		43.1 (7.0)	42.5 (8.7)	41.7 (7.5)	42.8 (8.8)	44.7 (8.0)	0.804
Equivalent	3.1 (1.1)	3.0 (1.2)	3.5 (0.9)	0.044		3.4 (0.9)	3.1 (1.1)	3.0 (1.2)	3.1 (1.1)	3.5 (1.1)	0.638
Failed	2 (2%)	2 (3.1%)	0 (0%)			0 (0%)	0 (0%)	1 (2.3%)	0 (0%)	1 (6.7%)	
Borderline	9 (9%)	8 (12.3%)	1 (2.9%)			0 (0%)	2 (14.3%)	5 (11.6%)	2 (12.5%)	0 (0%)	
Rey's delayed recall											
Corrected	8.7 (2.9)	8.2 (2.9)	9.5 (2.7)	0.03		9.5 (2.7)	9.0 (2.8)	8.1 (2.9)	8.4 (3.1)	9.6 (2.8)	0.327
Equivalen	3.0 (1.3)	2.8 (1.3)	3.3 (1.2)	0.03		3.3 (1.2)	3.0 (1.5)	2.8 (1.3)	2.7 (1.4)	3.3 (1.2)	0.58
Failed	7 (7%)	6 (9.2%)	1 (2.9%)			0 (0%)	1 (7.1%)	4 (9.3%)	1 (6.2%)	1 (6.7%)	
Borderline	10 (10%)	6 (9.2%)	4 (11.4%)			2 (16.7%)	2 (14.3%)	3 (7%)	3 (18.8%)	0 (0%)	
MFTC											
Time corrected	50.8 (31.7)	51.4 (25.5)	49.7 (41.3)	0.797		44.4 (26.7)	58.4 (26.1)	48.6 (36.4)	46.9 (25.4)	59.3 (32.5)	0.522
Time equivalent	3.8 (0.8)	3.8 (0.6)	3.6 (1.0)	0.133		3.6 (1.0)	3.6 (0.9)	3.8 (0.7)	3.9 (0.3)	3.7 (1.0)	0.703
Failed	2 (2%)	1 (1.5%)	1 (2.9%)			0 (0%)	0 (0%)	1 (2.3%)	0 (0%)	1 (6.7%)	
Borderline	2 (2%)	0 (0%)	2 (5.7%)			1 (8.3%)	1 (7.1%)	0 (0%)	0 (0%)	0 (0%)	
False alarms corrected	0.7 (2.5)	0.6 (2.9)	0.7 (1.3)	0.858		2.6 (6.4)	0.8 (1.9)	0.4 (1.0)	0.2 (0.8)	0.3 (0.8)	0.651
False alarms equivalent	3.5 (1.1)	3.7 (0.9)	3.2 (1.4)	0.042		2.8 (1.8)	3.4 (1.2)	3.6 (0.9)	3.7 (1.0)	3.7 (1.0)	0.149

Failed	7 (7%)	3 (4.6%)	4 (11.4%)		3 (25%)	1 (7.1%)	1 (2.3%)	1 (6.2%)	1 (6.7%)	
Borderline	2 (2%)	1 (1.5%)	1 (2.9%)		0 (0%)	0 (0%)	2 (4.7%)	0 (0%)	0 (0%)	
Frontal Assessment Battery										
Corrected	15.8 (1.9)	15.9 (1.8)	15.7 (2.1)	0.717	16.1 (2.2)	15.6 (2.0)	15.9 (1.9)	15.9 (1.1)	15.6 (2.2)	0.952
Equivalent	2.8 (1.4)	2.9 (1.4)	2.7 (1.5)	0.556	2.8 (1.6)	2.8 (1.4)	2.8 (1.4)	2.9 (1.1)	2.6 (1.8)	0.978
Failed	12 (12%)	6 (9.2%)	6 (17.1%)		2 (16.7%)	2 (14.3%)	4 (9.3%)	0 (0%)	4 (26.7%)	
Borderline	8 (8%)	7 (10.8%)	1 (2.9%)		1 (8.3%)	0 (0%)	5 (11.6%)	2 (12.5%)	0 (0%)	
Digit Span Forward										
Corrected	6.0 (1.1)	6.0 (1.1)	5.9 (1.1)	0.444	5.8 (0.9)	5.8 (1.1)	6.0 (1.1)	6.2 (1.2)	6.0 (1.0)	0.918
Equivalent	3.2 (1.3)	3.2 (1.2)	3.1 (1.4)	0.479	3.2 (1.3)	2.9 (1.6)	3.2 (1.3)	3.4 (1.3)	3.1 (1.1)	0.917
Failed	8 (8%)	4 (6.2%)	4 (11.4%)		1 (8.3%)	2 (14.3%)	4 (9.3%)	1 (6.2%)	0 (0%)	
Borderline	4 (4%)	3 (4.6%)	1 (2.9%)		0 (0%)	1 (7.1%)	1 (2.3%)	1 (6.2%)	1 (6.7%)	
Digit Span Backwards										
Corrected	4.1 (1.0)	4.2 (1.0)	3.9 (1.0)	0.26	4.3 (0.8)	4.0 (0.8)	4.1 (1.0)	3.8 (0.9)	4.1 (1.1)	0.701
Equivalent	2.7 (1.3)	2.8 (1.3)	2.5 (1.4)	0.279	3.1 (1.2)	2.6 (1.2)	2.8 (1.4)	2.6 (1.5)	2.6 (1.4)	0.852
Failed	8 (8%)	4 (6.2%)	4 (11.4%)		0 (0%)	0 (0%)	5 (11.6%)	2 (12.5%)	1 (6.7%)	
Borderline	15 (15%)	8 (12.3%)	7 (20%)		2 (16.7%)	3 (21.4%)	4 (9.3%)	3 (18.8%)	3 (20%)	
Trail Making										
Corrected	118.2 (100.6)	93.9 (86.8)	163.5 (109.7)	<.001	185.2 (121.7)	94.3 (91.1)	112.2 (99.2)	98.4 (89.8)	125.5 (94.8)	0.136
Equivalent	2.3 (1.5)	2.7 (1.4)	1.6 (1.5)	<.001	1.5 (1.7)	2.9 (1.5)	2.4 (1.6)	2.4 (1.4)	2.1 (1.4)	0.231
Failed	21 (21%)	8 (12.3%)	13 (37.1%)		6 (50%)	2 (14.3%)	8 (18.6%)	2 (12.5%)	3 (20%)	
Borderline	11 (11%)	7 (10.8%)	4 (11.4%)		0 (0%)	0 (0%)	6 (14%)	3 (18.8%)	2 (13.3%)	

Abbreviations: ECMO, extracorporeal membrane oxygenation; HFNC, high-flow nasal cannulae; MFTC, Multiple Features Target Cancellation test; MMSE, Mini Mental State Exam.

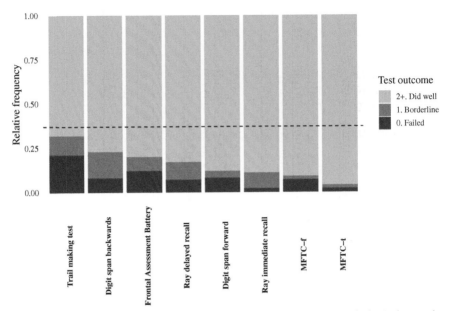

Fig. 2. Neuropsychological tests. The figure shows, for each neuropsychological test, the proportion of patients with fair (*light color*), borderline (*darker color*) or failed (*dark color*) outcome. Equivalent scores (ES) were used to rate participants: those with a score of 2 or more, 1, or zero were classified as having normal, borderline or pathologic performance respectively. Horizontal dashed line indicates the overall prevalence of participants classified as having a pathologic neuropsychological test (ie, ≥1 ES of zero and ≥1 ES of 1) MFTC, Multiple Features Target Cancellation test.

When directly tested with the neuropsychological battery, 33%, 23%, and 20% of participants failed the Trial Making, Digit Span Backwards, and Frontal Evaluation Battery tests, respectively, showing impairment in visuoperceptual skills, selective and divided attention, working memory, short-term verbal memory, and executive functions. These data expand the preliminary knowledge acquired in 2 previous studies with evidence of attention deficit,[29] visuoperception, naming, and fluency.[30]

An important finding from the study is that approximately 1 in 3 participants presented at neuropsychological tests with at least 1 overtly pathologic score in conjunction with at least 1 borderline pathologic test. This finding, together with average Mini Mental State Exam scores above the cutoff of 23 could represent a rough estimate of post–COVID-19 mild cognitive impairment. Such a value does not differ from that obtained in other studies based on telephone interviews.[31]

This study had many methodological limitations owing to the design and circumstances under which it was conducted. It is a single-center study with no control group or longitudinal follow-up. In addition, after an initial phase in which people were contacted from the hospital's patient lists, later people from the local area began to request to be followed at our center. Therefore, it is not possible to exclude that people with a greater burden of disease were included. Importantly no premorbid neuropsychological evaluation was available. Indeed, the sole use of neuropsychological tests could have inaccurately estimated the problem because an unknown proportion of participants could have presented pathologic performance on tests, regardless of COVID-19.

SUMMARY

COVID-19 is capable of eliciting persistent neurocognitive alterations. These alterations are measurable with widely available test batteries and seem particularly relevant in the areas of executive functions in general and attention and working memory specifically. In the context of this ongoing pandemic, it is imperative to intensify and expand research in the field as these cognitive derangements may represent an early stage of mild cognitive impairment in the elderly.

CLINICS CARE POINTS

- For many elderly people, Covid-19 represents an event with non-negligible cognitive sequelae.
- Since in many cases these people have never been previously studied cognitively, the clinician is confronted with the question of whether what is being observed is a more or less temporary effect of Covid-19 or on the contrary represents the onset of a cognitive impairment of a different nature although possibly triggered or made more readily apparent by Covid-19.
- In this sensitive population group, therefore, we recommend to proactively look for emerging cognitive deficits and to plan a reassessment of the cognitive picture at regular intervals.

SUPPLEMENTARY DATA

Supplementary data related to this article can be found online at https://doi.org/10.1016/j.cger.2022.05.003.

REFERENCES

1. Nalbandian A, Sehgal K, Gupta A, et al. Post-acute COVID-19 syndrome. Nat Med 2021. https://doi.org/10.1038/s41591-021-01283-z.
2. Carfì A, Bernabei R, Landi F. Persistent symptoms in patients after acute COVID-19. JAMA 2020;324(6):603.
3. Huang C, Huang L, Wang Y, et al. 6-month consequences of COVID-19 in patients discharged from hospital: a cohort study. Lancet 2021;397(10270):220–32.
4. Janiri D, Carfì A, Kotzalidis GD, et al. Posttraumatic stress disorder in patients after severe COVID-19 infection. JAMA Psychiatry 2021. https://doi.org/10.1001/jamapsychiatry.2021.0109.
5. Taquet M, Luciano S, Geddes JR, et al. Bidirectional associations between COVID-19 and psychiatric disorder: retrospective cohort studies of 62 354 COVID-19 cases in the USA. Lancet Psychiatry 2021;8(2):130–40.
6. Graham EL, Clark JR, Orban ZS, et al. Persistent neurologic symptoms and cognitive dysfunction in non-hospitalized Covid-19 "long haulers. Ann Clin Translational Neurol 2021. https://doi.org/10.1002/acn3.51350.
7. Tenforde MW, Kim SS, Lindsell CJ, et al. Symptom duration and risk factors for delayed return to usual health among[1] M. W. Tenforde et al., "Symptom duration and risk factors for delayed return to usual health among outpatients with COVID-19 in a multistate health care systems network — United. MMWR Morbidity Mortality Weekly Rep 2020;69(30):993–8.

8. Gemelli Against COVID-19 Post-Acute Care Study Group. Post-COVID-19 global health strategies: the need for an interdisciplinary approach. Aging Clin Exp Res 2020;32(8):1613–20.

9. Folstein MF, Folstein SE, McHugh PR. Mini-mental state". A practical method for grading the cognitive state of patients for the clinician. J Psychiatr Res 1975; 12(3):189–98.

10. Carlesimo GA, Sabbadini M, Fadda L, et al. Different components in word-list forgetting of pure amnesics, degenerative demented and healthy subjects. Cortex 1995;31(4):735–45.

11. Gainotti G, Marra C, Villa G. A double dissociation between accuracy and time of execution on attentional tasks in Alzheimer's disease and multi-infarct dementia. Brain 2001;124(Pt 4):731–8.

12. Standardizzazione e taratura italiana di test neuropsicologici. In: Spinnler H, Tognoni G, editors. Iialian J Neurol Sci 1987;8(6):120.

13. Giovagnoli AR, Del Pesce M, Mascheroni S, et al. Trail making test: normative values from 287 normal adult controls. Ital J Neurol Sci 1996;17(4):305–9.

14. Bowie CR, Harvey PD. Administration and interpretation of the trail making test. Nat Protoc 2006;1(5):2277–81.

15. Monaco M, Costa A, Caltagirone C, et al. Forward and backward span for verbal and visuo-spatial data: standardization and normative data from an Italian adult population. Neurol Sci 2013;34(5):749–54.

16. Dubois B, Slachevsky A, Litvan I, et al. The FAB: a frontal assessment battery at bedside. Neurology 2000;55(11):1621–6.

17. Appollonio I, Leone M, Isella V, et al. The Frontal Assessment Battery (FAB): normative values in an Italian population sample. Neurol Sci 2005;26(2):108–16.

18. Capitani E, Laiacona M. Composite neuropsychological batteries and demographic correction: standardization based on equivalent scores, with a review of published data. The Italian Group for the Neuropsychological Study of Ageing. J Clin Exp Neuropsychol 1997;19(6):795–809.

19. Hamilton M. The assessment of anxiety states by rating. Br J Med Psychol 1959; 32(1):50–5.

20. Maier W, Buller R, Philipp M, et al. The Hamilton Anxiety Scale: reliability, validity and sensitivity to change in anxiety and depressive disorders. J Affect Disord 1988;14(1):61–8.

21. Hamilton M. A rating scale for depression. J Neurol Neurosurg Psychiatry 1960; 23:56–62.

22. Zimmerman M, Martinez JH, Young D, et al. Severity classification on the Hamilton depression rating scale. J Affect Disord 2013;150(2):384–8.

23. Andrews G, Slade T. Interpreting scores on the Kessler Psychological Distress scale (K10). Aust N Z J Public Health 2001;25(6):494–7.

24. Kessler RC, Andrews G, Colpe LJ, et al. Short screening scales to monitor population prevalences and trends in non-specific psychological distress. Psychol Med 2002;32(6):959–76.

25. Buysse DJ, Reynolds CF, Monk TH, et al. The Pittsburgh Sleep Quality Index: a new instrument for psychiatric practice and research. Psychiatry Res 1989; 28(2):193–213.

26. Cao B, Wang Y, Wen D, et al. A trial of lopinavir-ritonavir in adults hospitalized with severe Covid-19. N Engl J Med 2020;382(19):1787–99.

27. Scully EP, Haverfield J, Ursin RL, et al. Considering how biological sex impacts immune responses and COVID-19 outcomes. Nat Rev Immunol 2020;20(7):442–7.

28. Huang C, Wang Y, Li X, et al. Clinical features of patients infected with 2019 novel coronavirus in Wuhan, China. Lancet 2020;395(10223):497–506.
29. Zhou H, Lu S, Chen J, et al. The landscape of cognitive function in recovered COVID-19 patients. J Psychiatr Res 2020;129(January):98–102.
30. Amalakanti S, Arepalli KVR, Jillella JP. Cognitive assessment in asymptomatic COVID-19 subjects. VirusDisease 2021. https://doi.org/10.1007/s13337-021-00663-w. Mci).
31. Liu YH, Chen Y, Wang QH, et al. One-year trajectory of cognitive changes in older survivors of COVID-19 in Wuhan, China: a longitudinal cohort study. JAMA Neurol 2022. https://doi.org/10.1001/JAMANEUROL.2022.0461.

COVID-19 Vaccines in Older Adults

Challenges in Vaccine Development and Policy Making

Chih-Kuang Liang, MD, PhD[a,b], Wei-Ju Lee, MD, PhD[a,c],
Li-Ning Peng, MD, PhD[a,d], Lin-Chieh Meng, BS Pharm[e],
Fei-Yuan Hsiao, PhD[e,f,g], Liang-Kung Chen, MD, PhD[a,d,h],*

KEYWORDS

• COVID-19 • Disability • Frailty • Immunosenescence • Vaccine

KEY POINTS

- Older adults are a vulnerable group with a high need for coronavirus disease 2019 (COVID-19) vaccines, but these individuals are also more prone to the development of vaccine-related adverse events.
- Older adults with frailty, disability, dementia or living in long-term care facilities need special attention in COVID-19 vaccination programs because supporting evidence for the safety and efficacy of COVID-19 vaccines in these individuals is limited.
- The active involvement of geriatricians in vaccine development and related public-policy development is important for the success of adult vaccination strategies against COVID-19 and other communicable and noncommunicable diseases.
- The completion of a primary series of COVID-19 vaccines with a heterologous booster dose remains the best strategy to reduce the impact of severe acute respiratory syndrome coronavirus-2 (SARS-CoV-2) infections and transmission.

[a] Center for Healthy Longevity and Aging Sciences, National Yang Ming Chiao Tung University, Taipei, Taiwan; [b] Center for Geriatrics and Gerontology, Kaohsiung Veterans General Hospital, Kaohsiung, Taiwan; [c] Department of Family Medicine, Taipei Veterans General Hospital Yuanshan Branch, Yi-Lan, Taiwan; [d] Center for Geriatrics and Gerontology, Taipei Veterans General Hospital, Taipei, Taiwan; [e] Graduate Institute of Clinical Pharmacy, College of Medicine, National Taiwan University, Taipei, Taiwan; [f] School of Pharmacy, College of Medicine, National Taiwan University, Taipei, Taiwan; [g] Department of Pharmacy, National Taiwan University, Taipei, Taiwan; [h] Taipei Municipal Gan-Dau Hospital (Managed by Taipei Veterans General Hospital), Taipei, Taiwan
* Corresponding author. Center for Geriatrics and Gerontology, Taipei Veterans General Hospital, No. 201, Sec 2, Shih-Pai Road, Taipei, Taiwan
E-mail address: lkchen2@vghtpe.gov.tw

Clin Geriatr Med 38 (2022) 605–620
https://doi.org/10.1016/j.cger.2022.03.006
0749-0690/22/© 2022 Elsevier Inc. All rights reserved.

geriatric.theclinics.com

INTRODUCTION

Coronavirus disease 2019 (COVID-19), caused by severe acute respiratory syndrome coronavirus 2 (SARS-CoV-2), was first reported in December 2019 and was declared a global pandemic on March 11, 2020, by the World Health Organization (WHO). By the end of 2021, there were 288,306,329 confirmed cases and 5,438,835 COVID-19–related deaths according to the WHO Coronavirus Dashboard.[1] The COVID-19 pandemic has substantially affected health care systems and societies across the world, and this impact will last longer than expected. Public health crises such as the COVID-19 pandemic and extreme weather have strong adverse impacts on vulnerable populations, such as children, the disadvantaged, frail older adults, and people with disability or dementia.[2–5] Studies have clearly shown the vulnerability of these populations when encountering a public health crisis (eg, earthquakes, extreme weather, and pandemics), and special attention and care plans are needed to tackle these challenges.[6] Older people are generally considered a high-risk population in clinical services because they are more likely to present atypical symptoms, multimorbidity, geriatric syndromes, functional limitations, and unexpected clinical outcomes.[7,8] The knowledge and clinical experiences in the treatment of older people with acute illnesses can be applied to the COVID-19 pandemic. A recent systematic review and meta-analysis included 13,624 older patients with COVID-19 and identified that approximately half of older patients with COVID-19 had severe illness, one-fifth were critically ill, and one-tenth died.[9] Because of their high disease severity and mortality risk, older people have become the priority in COVID-19 vaccination programs.

The success of COVID-19 vaccine development, together with extensive global public health efforts (face masks, hand hygiene, lockdowns, and many others), brought a glimmer of hope to the control of the COVID-19 pandemic. All countries started their vaccination plans based on the availability and access to COVID-19 vaccines, and most countries prioritized older adults and nursing home residents for vaccination because of their high risk of severe illness and mortality.[10] However, the vaccination strategies also caused some unexpected challenges, because potential vaccine-related deaths negatively influenced the willingness of many people to receive COVID-19 vaccines.[11,12] The challenges of COVID-19 vaccination in older adults involve many different issues, including multimorbidity, frailty, disability, and immunosenescence (a process of immune dysfunction that occurs with age and inflammaging), which are all important factors for COVID-19 severity, complications, and the effectiveness of vaccines.[13] Nevertheless, the proportion of older adults included in the available vaccine clinical trials is usually low. For example, only 24.8% of participants in the Moderna vaccine trial were people aged 65 years and older,[14] and only 5% of participants in the Oxford-AstraZeneca trial were people aged 70 years and older.[15] The safety, efficacy, and vaccination strategies of COVID-19 vaccines in older adults, especially frail older people, have not been well researched. Therefore, this review focuses on the challenges of COVID-19 vaccines and related policy development in older adults, with a special focus on those with frailty, disability, dementia, or living in nursing homes.

CHALLENGES OF VACCINATIONS IN OLDER ADULTS

Although vaccinations have become one of the most widely accepted preventive services in the world, and older adults, as a vulnerable population, need those preventive services most, they are also susceptible to vaccine-related adverse effects.[16] Despite all safety and efficacy concerns, vaccination remains a cost-effective approach to reduce the burden of communicable and associated noncommunicable conditions.

Experiences in vaccinations in older adults may provide some insights for COVID-19 vaccine and policy development. The development of vaccines to prevent viral infections or disease reactivation in older adults, such as influenza or herpes zoster, has shown that older adults with frailty, disability, dementia, or living in nursing homes are more susceptible to vaccine-related adverse events, and the risks may sometimes outweigh the clinical benefits.[17]

The immune systems of older people differ greatly from those of young adults and middle-aged people, especially cellular immunity, so the immunogenicity and efficacy of vaccines usually remain questionable in older people with frailty, disability, and dementia. Most vaccines used in older people are less immunogenic and effective than those used in younger adults,[18] which results from several factors, such as immunosenescence, inflammation, and altered immune responses to infections and vaccines.[19] Hence, older people need special attention in vaccine development. For example, influenza virus is transmitted via direct contact, droplets, and fomites, and particularly increases the burden of disease and mortality in those aged 75 years and older.[20,21] However, the effectiveness of influenza vaccine was found to be only approximately 29% to 48% in elderly individuals.[22] The reduced vaccine effectiveness results in a lower prevention rate of hospital admissions due to influenza among older adults (37%; 95% confidence interval [CI], 30%–44%) than among younger adults aged 18 to 64 years (51%; 95% CI, 44%–58%).[23] However, the effectiveness of influenza vaccine to prevent any influenza-associated deaths was shown to be well preserved (74%; 95% CI, 44.0%–88.4%) for people aged 65 years and older.[24] The reduced vaccine effectiveness in older adults is related to several factors, such as the virus strain, vaccination rates, seasonal factors, geographic demography, infection history, and frailty or multimorbidity. Despite all the factors mentioned earlier, older age is a key player in vaccine effectiveness.[25]

Current strategies to enhance vaccine immunogenicity and efficacy in older adults include increasing the vaccine dose or adding appropriate adjuvants to trigger immunostimulation, which are common in vaccine development for older people.[21,22] A previous meta-analysis suggested that a high-dose influenza vaccine was consistently more effective than a standard-dose influenza vaccine in reducing influenza cases and influenza-associated clinical complications.[26] In addition, the recombinant influenza vaccine using DNA recombination technology to produce influenza hemagglutinin protein in the cell culture instead of growing live influenza virus in embryos has been developed with success. Recombinant influenza vaccines also included high-dose vaccines (3 times the influenza antigens). All 3 types of enhanced influenza vaccines mentioned earlier induced higher antibody responses than standard-dose vaccines, maintained improvements in immunogenicity, and had better protection in people aged more than 75 years and those with chronic diseases (heart or lung conditions).[22]

Similarly, the effects of immune aging have been observed in herpes zoster vaccines. The live, attenuated herpes zoster vaccine was the first vaccine developed for herpes zoster prevention, and it significantly and safely increased varicella zoster virus–specific T cell–mediated immunity (51.3% effective rate in preventing herpes zoster; 66.5% effective rate in preventing postherpetic neuralgia).[27] However, the effectiveness of the herpes zoster vaccine was significantly affected by age. The Shingles Prevention Study[27] demonstrated that the live, attenuated zoster vaccine reduced the herpes zoster burden of illness by 61.1% (65.5% in subjects aged 60–69 years; 55.4% in subjects aged ≥70 years), the incidence of clinically significant postherpetic neuralgia by 66.5% (65.7% in subjects aged 60–69 years; 66.8% in subjects aged ≥70 years), and the incidence of herpes zoster by 51.3% (63.9% in subjects aged 60–69 years, but only 37.6% in subjects aged $\geq$70 years).[28] Another vaccine against herpes zoster is the recombinant subunit herpes zoster vaccine, which consists of recombinant varicella zoster virus glycoprotein E and the AS01B adjuvant system. Varicella zoster virus glycoprotein E is the most abundant glycoprotein in cells infected with varicella zoster virus and thus becomes the main target of varicella zoster virus–specific antibodies and T cells.[29] AS01B adjuvant systems included 2 types of adjuvants, 3-O-desacyl-4'-monophosphoryl lipid A (MPL) and QS-21, which stimulate virus glycoprotein E–specific CD4+ T cell and antibody responses in animal models.[30] The pooled efficacy of the recombinant subunit herpes zoster vaccine was 91.3%, and the vaccine efficacy was similar across ages ranging from 50 to 59 years, 60 to 69 years, and 70 years and older.[31,32] The experiences in herpes zoster vaccine development were similar to those of influenza vaccines and thus may become common challenges in the development of vaccines for older people.

In pneumococcal vaccination, currently, the 23-valent pneumococcal polysaccharide vaccine against *Streptococcus pneumoniae* (PPV23) has been replaced by a 13-valent conjugated pneumococcal vaccine (PCV13).[33] PPV23 successfully induced immunity in older adults against pneumococcal diseases, but the protective effects declined over time. Despite the declining efficacy of PPV23 in older adults, the booster dose of PPV23 was not recommended for various reasons. PCV13 was originally developed for young children to overcome the limitations of T cell–independent polysaccharide antigens, but it protects against pneumonia only approximately 50% of the time.[34] In 2019, the United States Advisory Committee on Immunization Practice removed the recommendation for routine PCV13 use among people aged 65 years and older. In contrast, routine 1-dose PPV23 use for people aged 65 years and older remains in the recommendations, and only those individuals at risk for exposure to PCV13 serotypes are recommended to receive PCV13 vaccinations.[35] If the decision is made to administer a PCV13 vaccine, it should be administered at least 1 year before a PPV23 vaccine. The use of pneumococcal vaccines also reflects the challenges in vaccination for older adults because of the clinical characteristics, immune responses, personal risks in the life course, and the efficacy of vaccines in this population.

CORONAVIRUS DISEASE 2019 VACCINE DEVELOPMENT

The success of COVID-19 vaccine development has been widely recognized as an important key to ending the pandemic. To date, several different platforms of technology have been used to develop COVID-19 vaccines, including DNA, messenger RNA (mRNA), nonreplicating viral vector, protein subunit, and inactivated vaccines.[36–39] Each COVID-19 vaccine platform has its own unique advantages and disadvantages based on cultivation technology, production speed, large-scale production, vaccine safety, storage and transportation requirements, and the effectiveness of the immune response triggered (**Table 1**).

Protein-based vaccines account for the largest proportion of COVID-19 vaccine development (35.9%).[40] The latest update at the end of 2021 showed that the WHO has approved 10 COVID-19 vaccines from 8 original vaccines based on 4 vaccine technological platforms (mRNA, nonreplicating viral vector, inactivated vaccine, and protein subunit platforms).[36,40,41] Recombinant viral vector vaccines consist of replicating and nonreplicating types based on their ability to replicate in host cells. The adenoviral (Ad) vector is the most commonly used viral vector. A safe viral vector is a delivery system that contains antigens and molecules that can induce both

Table 1
Overview of the characteristics of major vaccine technology platforms and vaccines used to prevent severe acute respiratory syndrome coronavirus-2 infections

	Vaccine Platform	Existing Vaccine Examples Approved by the WHO[36,37]	Production Speed[36,37]	Immune Response[36,37]	Advantages[36–39]	Disadvantages[36–39]
Traditional approaches	Live, attenuated	• Under development	Slow	Both cellular and humoral	• Broad antigenic profile • Strong and long-lasting immune response	• Safety issues in immunocompromised and pregnant people • Require dedicated biosafety facilities • Can be complicated to scale up manufacturing
	Inactivated	• Covaxin (Bharat Biotech (India)) • Covilo (Sinopharm (Beijing)) • CoronaVac (Sinovac (China))	Medium	Mostly humoral	• Broad antigenic profile • Safe • Convenient transport and storage	• Reduced immune response • Risk of vaccine-enhanced disease • Antibody titers reduce over time • Requirement for biosafety facilities • Lower purity
	Protein subunit	• Nuvaxovid (Novavax) • COVOVAX (Serum Institute of India [Novavax formulation]) • MVC-COV1901 (Medigen)[a]	Medium	Humoral	• Safe for immunocompromised people • Noninfectious • Simple and less expensive to produce • Targeting key antigens	• Limited capability in inducing cellular immunity • Unstable structure, which may lead to a loss of immunogenicity • Several booster doses and adjuvants are often needed • Challenges in large-scale production
Novel approaches	Viruslike particles	• Under development	Medium	Both cellular and humoral	• Noninfectious • Broad antigenic profile • Safe • Scalability of production	• Limited immunogenicity • Lower purity
	Nonreplicating viral vector	• Ad26.COV2.S (Janssen	Medium	Both cellular and humoral	• Fast to produce • Reusable platform	• Preexisting immunity against the vector

(continued on next page)

Table 1
(*continued*)

Vaccine Platform	Existing Vaccine Examples Approved by the WHO[36,37]	Production Speed[36,37]	Immune Response[36,37]	Advantages[36-39]	Disadvantages[36-39]
	• [Johnson & Johnson]) • Vaxzevria (Oxford/AstraZeneca) • Covishield (Serum Institute of India [Oxford/AstraZeneca formulation])			• Safe • Strong immune response	• Risk of adverse reactions
Replicating viral vector	• Under development	Fast	Both cellular and humoral	• Fast to produce • Lower doses/single dose • Reusable platform • Strong immune response • Less infectious	• Preexisting immunity against the vector • Risk of adverse reactions
DNA	• Under development	Fast	Both cellular and humoral	• Fast to produce • Robust immune response • Scalable • Noninfectious • Reusable platform • Stable at room temperature	• May need special devices for storage and transport • No DNA-based vaccine has previously been produced • Potential genome integration risk
mRNA	• Spikevax (Moderna) • Comirnaty (Pfizer/BioNTech)	Fast	Both cellular and humoral	• Fast to produce • Strong immune response • Noninfectious • No genome integration risk • Reusable platform • Stimulates strong T-cell response • Simple formulations	• May need extremely low temperatures for storage and transportation • No mRNA-based vaccine has previously been produced

[a] Not approved by WHO until 31 January 2022 (https://covid19.trackvaccines.org/agency/who/) but has been recommended by an independent vaccine prioritization advisory group to be included in the WHO Solidarity Trial Vaccines (STv).

antibody-mediated and cell-mediated immune responses. After invading the host cells, the antigen gene is inserted into the nucleus of the host cells, and the viral protein is produced on the surface of the host cells to induce host immune responses. Inactivated vaccines contain completely inactivated or killed pathogens (a part of the killed pathogen or the whole pathogen) and primarily induce protective antibodies against epitopes on hemagglutinin glycoprotein on the surface of the virus. Compared with live, attenuated vaccines, inactivated vaccines usually induce a weaker immune response, so an adjuvant is usually needed to increase the effectiveness of the immune response. The manufacturing principles of recombinant protein-based (protein subunit) vaccines are to identify the required pathogenic protein from the virus coat, implant the DNA sequence for the target protein into a cell culture, and purify the target protein for the vaccines. The human immune system detects the viral protein when the vaccine is injected and generates an immune response against future infections. Protein-based vaccines are generally safe because they contain noninfectious protein subunits and induce sufficient antibody-mediated immune responses, but they also need adjuvants to induce long-lasting immune responses. The mRNA vaccines include mRNA molecules encoding antigens to induce target protein production without affecting the DNA of host cells. The mRNA vaccine is composed of mRNA encapsulated in lipid nanoparticles, which protects the RNA structure and facilitates host cell absorption. After the mRNA vaccine is injected into muscle, the cells translate it into spike proteins. The produced spike proteins further emerge on the surface of cell membranes and are secreted into body fluids for immunostimulation.

Two mRNA-based COVID-19 vaccines were approved for emergency use authorization (EUA) by the US FDA on 11 December 2020 (BNT162b2) and 18 December 2020 (mRNA-1273) to control the COVID-19 pandemic.[36–39] BNT162b2 is an mRNA-based vaccine encoding the SARS-CoV-2 receptor binding domain that was jointly developed by BioNTech in Germany and Pfizer in the United States. BNT162b2 is a lipid nanoparticle–formulated, nucleoside-modified RNA vaccine that works against the S protein of the SARS-CoV-2. The mRNA in BNT162b2 encodes a SARS-CoV-2 full-length spike protein modified by 2 proline mutations to ensure that the protein remains in the prefusion conformation. BNT162b2 was approved by the WHO on 31 December 2020 and has been approved in 122 countries.[42] mRNA-1273, another mRNA-based vaccine developed by Moderna, was approved by the WHO on 30 April 2021 and has been approved in 83 countries.[42] The mRNA-1273 vaccine contains a lipid nanoparticle-encapsulated nucleoside-modified mRNA that encodes the full-length spike protein of SARS-CoV-2, S(2P), a prefusion protein that is stabilized after replacing S protein residues 986 and 987 with the 2P mutation. The spike glycoprotein is the primary vaccine target, because it is essential for the virus to attach and enter host cells. mRNA-1273 triggers a neutralizing antibody response and eliminates the virus by inducing CD4+ T cell and CD8+ cytotoxic T-cell responses.[43,44]

CORONAVIRUS DISEASE 2019 VACCINE ACCEPTANCE

Although COVID-19 vaccines are an effective strategy to control the COVID-19 pandemic, a significant proportion of people refuse COVID-19 vaccination, even though the benefits of vaccinations have been clearly demonstrated. A global survey of potential acceptance of COVID-19 vaccines from 19 countries in mid-2020 showed that 71.5% of participants reported positive attitudes toward COVID-19 vaccination (ranging from 65.2% in Sweden to 88.6% in China).[45] However, another systematic review included data from 33 countries at the end of 2020 and identified high variability in COVID-19 vaccine acceptance rates across countries.[46] COVID-19 vaccine acceptance rates were particularly low in the Middle East, Eastern Europe, and Russia (<60%). In contrast, high acceptance rates were noted in east and southeast Asia (>90%).[46] It was estimated that a 60% to 75% vaccination rate of all populations is needed to slow or stop the transmission and community spreading of COVID-19.[47–49] In the older population, the vaccination rate is higher than that in adults or younger populations. In the United States, approximately 99.9% and 98.1% of older adults aged 65 to 74 and 75 years and older, respectively, have received at least 1 dose of a COVID-19 vaccine, and 89.7% and 84.4% of them were fully vaccinated. However, only 74.6% and 82.7% of people aged 25 to 39 and 40 to 49 years have received at least 1 dose of a COVID-19 vaccine.[50] In the United Kingdom, nearly 95% of older adults aged 65 years old and older have received a full dose of a COVID-19 vaccine.[51]

To improve the overall vaccination rates to increase herd immunity against COVID-19, it is important to explore vaccine acceptance in different regions and the reasons for rejection. A systematic review of 15 studies found that ethnicity, working status, religiosity, politics, sex, age, education, and income status were all predisposing factors to accept or refuse COVID-19 vaccination.[52] The most common reasons to decline COVID-19 vaccination were attitudes against vaccinations in general, concerns about safety because of the short development process, beliefs that vaccines were unnecessary because of the harmless nature of COVID-19, general distrust, doubt about the provenience of vaccines, and a lack of faith in vaccine efficacy.[53,54] In addition, the limited number of older individuals in clinical trials is a strong reason to reject COVID-19 vaccination because these individuals are at high risk for severe illness and vaccine-related adverse events.[55] Older adults' decisions for COVID-19 vaccination, especially for those with cognitive impairment, physical disability, frailty, and/or low sociocultural status, may be influenced by their family members or peers. Limited access to facilities for vaccinations is another obstacle for frail older adults to receive COVID-19 vaccines. A well-designed health care system and an effective public health system are critical to identify people in need and provide necessary services. In addition to compulsory measures, effective education and adequate information strategies for the target population are important to improve vaccination rates.[56]

CHALLENGES OF CORONAVIRUS DISEASE 2019 VACCINATION IN OLDER ADULTS

The successful development of COVID-19 vaccines has strengthened pandemic control strategies; the WHO aimed to achieve 70% vaccination coverage by mid-2022, and older people were prioritized for vaccination to reduce mortality, severe morbidity, and related hospitalizations.[57] Most countries prioritized older adults for COVID-19 vaccinations because of their vulnerability and susceptibility to infections.[58] The WHO published a framework to guide mass vaccination policies[59] and to encourage countries to publish and monitor the progress of their vaccination programs.[60] Hasan and colleagues[61] reviewed 15 national policies and summarized critical elements for successful vaccination policies, including equitable access and vaccination scheduling, vaccination locations, coordination with cold chain infrastructure, planning for staff for vaccinations, and community engagement to enhance the efficiency of vaccination strategies.[61] Among these strategies, the capacity to provide COVID-19 vaccinations is the most critical, and creating facilities for and access to mass COVID-19 vaccination should be the priority.[62] In many countries, locations such as large public venues, hospitals, clinics, pharmacies, and even malls are used to increase vaccination accessibility.[61] Incorporating routine vaccines such as influenza, pneumococcal, or herpes zoster vaccines with COVID-19 vaccines is also an effective approach.[63]

Despite the challenges in public policy for mass COVID-19 vaccination in older adults, special challenges related to the health characteristics of older adults remain. In real-world practice, frail older people or nursing home residents were earmarked as having first priority for COVID-19 immunization, but they were not included in any phase of the clinical trials of COVID-19 vaccine development.[64] A recent review of 12 COVID-19 therapeutic or prophylactic trials showed that the average age of enrolled participants was 20 years younger than the average age of participants in large observational studies, and none of those trials reported on cognitive performance or functional outcomes, the foremost determinants of the health of older people.[65] Concern regarding the underrepresentation of older or frail populations in the trials included that the validity of vaccines for these vulnerable groups may be compromised.[66] Although 42.2% of the Pfizer/BioNTech vaccine trial participants were aged 55 years old and older, less than 5% of individuals were older than 75 years.[67] Approximately one-quarter of Moderna vaccine trial participants were aged 65 years and older,[14] but the Oxford-AstraZeneca vaccine trial enrolled only 5% participants aged 70 years old and older.[15] The Oxford-AstraZeneca vaccine trial further excluded those with cognitive impairment and frailty,[15] the individuals potentially most susceptible to SARS-CoV-2 infections.[68] An observational study on a long-term care facility disclosed that SARS-CoV-2 infection-naive residents showed delayed, lower responses to COVID-19 vaccines, which were less effective in antagonizing the spike protein of viral variants.[69]

Because of the lack of evidence on the safety and efficacy in this special population, postmarket surveillance for COVID-19 vaccines is an important alternative to examine the safety and efficacy of these vaccines. The Norwegian government received 100 reports of suspected vaccine-related deaths after providing BNT162b2 mRNA vaccines for approximately 35,000 nursing home residents,[70] and 10 probable and 26 possible vaccine-related fatal events were concluded after careful cross-examinations by experts. The vaccine-related fatality risk may be related to the existing frailty and disability, instead of older age itself. However, public attention related to postvaccination deaths substantially increased the hesitancy of nursing home staff toward COVID-19 vaccination,[71] as well as the lay public. The vulnerable groups needing vaccines are also those susceptible to adverse reactions. A study reported the favorable effects of BNT162b2 mRNA COVID-19 vaccines in older adults with frailty or living in long-term care facilities,[72] but the small sample size (134 residents from 5 long-term care facilities) and inclusion criteria (58.2% participants infected by SARS-CoV-2) meant that concerns were not completely addressed. In particular, the study concluded that only previous SARS-CoV-2 infection status was associated with vaccine immunogenicity.

A large prospective cohort study based on more than 10,000 care home residents reported that COVID-19 vaccines (BNT162b2 and Oxford-AstraZeneca) significantly reduced the transmission of COVID-19 but did not eliminate the infection risk.[73] Because of the lack of well-designed research, a study used a mathematical model to examine the roles of vaccine coverage in nursing homes and showed that increasing vaccine coverage of the nursing home staff, not vaccination of the residents, was the key to reducing symptomatic cases among nursing home residents.[74] A study of 2501 nursing homes in the United States supported the results of this analysis and showed that vaccinations for both residents and care staff significantly reduced SARS-CoV-2 infections in both residents and nursing staff, especially in nursing homes with fewer certified beds and higher numbers of nursing staff.[75]

Although vaccinations did not entirely prevent postvaccination breakthrough SARS-CoV-2 infections, these breakthrough infections were mostly mild or asymptomatic.[76] More research efforts in COVID-19 vaccine development and vaccination strategies among older persons with frailty, disability, dementia, long-term care facility residence, or home-bound status are needed.[77]

Although the WHO and most countries emphasized the importance of increasing the coverage of primary vaccination series to control the COVID-19 pandemic, breakthrough infections by SARS-CoV-2 variants such as Delta or Omicron triggered the need for booster doses. A recent systematic review and meta-regression analysis showed that the average declines in vaccine effectiveness over 6 months for symptomatic COVID-19 and severe COVID-19 in all age groups were 25.4% and 8.0%, respectively.[78] In particular, among persons aged 50 years old and older, the vaccine effectiveness decreased by 32% for symptomatic COVID-19 and by 10% for severe COVID-19.[78] A booster dose is recommended for individuals who have completed their primary vaccination series because of waning vaccine effectiveness over time, as well as the threats from Omicron and Delta variants. In 2022, an updated revision of the WHO Strategic Advisory Group of Experts summarized 2 key findings to recommend a booster dose. First, within the priority-use group, increasing the primary vaccination series coverage rate had a greater impact on reducing hospitalizations and deaths per dose than the use of an equivalent vaccine supply to increase the booster-dose coverage rate. Second, across priority-use groups, increasing the booster-dose coverage rate for higher priority-use groups yielded greater reductions in severe disease and deaths than the use of an equivalent vaccine supply to increase the primary vaccination series coverage rates of lower priority-use groups.[79]

Although the optimal interval to administer the booster dose has yet to be determined, an interval of 4 to 6 months after the completion of the primary vaccination series is a widely accepted scheme. The next challenge for the booster dose is the choice of using homologous or heterologous vaccines. A phase 1/2, open-label clinical trial conducted at 10 sites in the United States compared the serial use of homologous and heterologous boosters of BNT162b2, mRNA-1273, and Ad26.COV2.S vaccines, and disclosed acceptable reactogenicity and humoral immunogenicity for all combinations except for spike-specific T-cell responses in the homologous Ad26.COV2.S-boosted subgroup.[80] Another study in the Netherlands also found that heterologous regimens significantly increased immunogenicity and reactogenicity compared with homologous regimens in health care workers who received the Ad26.COV2.S vaccine as the initial vaccine.[81] Compared with homologous booster groups, the heterologous booster groups showed superior responses of antispike immunoglobulin G antibodies 28 days after the booster dose among those who had received 2 doses of CoronaVac.[82] In addition, 2 studies also found that participants who received a booster dose of the BNT162b2 vaccine had significantly lower rates of SARS-CoV-2 infections and severe illness than those who did not receive a booster dose.[83,84] The WHO reviewed available evidence and recommended that either homologous or heterologous schedules should be used. They also provided 3 heterologous schedules of primary and booster vaccination series: (1) initial doses of inactivated vaccines, with vectored or mRNA vaccines considered for subsequent doses; (2) initial doses of vectored vaccines, with mRNA vaccines considered for subsequent doses; and (3) initial doses of mRNA vaccines, with vectored vaccines considered for subsequent doses. Similar to the WHO recommendation, the US government recommended an interval of at least 5 months for mRNA vaccine (BNT162b2 and mRNA-1273) boosters.[85] Specifically, a booster can be given at least 2 months after receiving a primary Ad26.COV2.S vaccine.

THE ROLE OF GERIATRICIANS IN VACCINE DEVELOPMENT AND POLICY MAKING

Older people with frailty, disability, dementia, or living in nursing homes need special attention during the COVID-19 pandemic because of their high risk of infections, severe illness, mortality, lower vaccine responses, and vaccine adverse events, as well as their reduced access to health care services, reduced daily activities, and adverse impacts from activity restriction and lockdowns.[86] Some unique issues for vaccine development, clinical trial designs, outcome measurements, safety issues, and postmarket surveillance should be addressed to improve vaccine development and related vaccination policy making.[87] Involving geriatricians in COVID-19 vaccine-development and policy-making processes is important because of the special health and socioeconomic characteristics of older people, especially those with frailty, disability, dementia, or living in nursing homes.[88] It may be argued that including frail older people in vaccine clinical trials may delay vaccine development because this would likely lead to poorer safety or efficacy profiles, but these individuals are usually the prioritized group for vaccination. With the active participation of geriatricians in the vaccine-development and policy-making processes, the clinical trial design may be modified to include certain subsamples to examine the safety and efficacy of COVID-19 vaccines in this vulnerable group, and the development of vaccination policies may be improved with input from these professionals.[64]

SUMMARY

The success of COVID-19 vaccine development through various technological platforms has substantially relieved the impacts of the COVID-19 pandemic, because COVID-19 vaccines not only have prevented COVID-19 transmission but also have reduced the rates of severe COVID-19 and mortality. Special attention to older adults with frailty, disability, or dementia or living in nursing homes is needed in vaccine development, clinical trial designs, and vaccination policies. Despite the abovementioned concerns, the completion of a primary series of COVID-19 vaccines with heterologous booster doses in intervals of 4 to 6 months remains the best strategy to reduce the impact of SARS-CoV-2 infections and to obtain immunity against COVID-19 transmission.

CLINICS CARE POINTS

- Older adults with frailty, disability, dementia, or living in nursing homes are vulnerable to SARS-CoV-2 infections, but are also susceptible to vaccine-related adverse events. More clinical attention should be paid and more thorough explanations should be provided to vaccinees and their families.

- Limited evidence confirms the safety and efficacy of COVID-19 vaccinations for frail older adults in long-term care settings, and all necessary infection controls should be maintained after vaccinations, especially the care staff in long-term care settings.

- The completion of a primary series of COVID-19 vaccines with heterologous booster dose in intervals of 4 to 6 months remains the best strategy to reduce the impact of SARS-CoV-2 infections and to obtain immunity against COVID-19 transmission.

- Active involvement of geriatricians in vaccine development and related public-policy development is important for the success of adult vaccination strategies against COVID-19.

ACKNOWLEDGMENTS

The authors would like to express gratitude to the staff of the Center for Healthy Longevity and Aging Sciences of National Yang Ming Chiao Tung University for all research assistance, the National Health Research Institutes for funding support (NHRI-11A1-CG-CO-01-2225-1), and all researchers dedicated to vaccine development. Moreover, the authors would like to express their condolences to the families of individuals who died of COVID-19 for their loss.

REFERENCES

1. WHO coronavirus disease (COVID-19) dashboard. World Health Organization. Available at. https://covid19.who.int/. Accessed January 28, 2022.
2. Mostaza JM, García-Iglesias F, González-Alegre T, et al. Clinical course and prognostic factors of COVID-19 infection in an elderly hospitalized population. Arch Gerontol Geriatr 2020;91:104204.
3. Rowe TA, Patel M, O'Conor R, et al. COVID-19 exposures and infection control among home care agencies. Arch Gerontol Geriatr 2020;91:104214.
4. Bernabeu-Wittel M, Ternero-Vega JE, Díaz-Jiménez P, et al. Death risk stratification in elderly patients with covid-19. A comparative cohort study in nursing homes outbreaks. Arch Gerontol Geriatr 2020;91:104240.
5. Pranata R, Huang I, Lim MA, et al. Delirium and mortality in coronavirus disease 2019 (COVID-19) - a systematic review and meta-analysis. Arch Gerontol Geriatr 2021;95:104388.
6. Ahmadi S, Khankeh H, Sahaf R, et al. How did older adults respond to challenges after an earthquake? results from a qualitative study in Iran. Arch Gerontol Geriatr 2018;77:189–95.
7. Gómez-Belda AB, Fernández-Garcés M, Mateo-Sanchis E, et al. COVID-19 in older adults: what are the differences with younger patients? Geriatr Gerontol Int 2021;21(1):60–5.
8. Chen LK. COVID-19 vaccination and frailty in older adults. Arch Gerontol Geriatr 2021;96:104487.
9. Singhal S, Kumar P, Singh S, et al. Clinical features and outcomes of COVID-19 in older adults: a systematic review and meta-analysis. BMC Geriatr 2021; 21(1):321.
10. Teo SP. Review of COVID-19 vaccines and their evidence in older adults. Ann Geriatr Med Res 2021;25(1):4–9.
11. Hara M, Ishibashi M, Nakane A, et al. Differences in COVID-19 vaccine acceptance, hesitancy, and confidence between healthcare workers and the general population in Japan. Vaccines (Basel) 2021;9(12):1389.
12. Gallant AJ, Nicholls LAB, Rasmussen S, et al. Changes in attitudes to vaccination as a result of the COVID-19 pandemic: a longitudinal study of older adults in the UK. PLoS One 2021;16(12):e0261844.
13. Chen LK. Older adults and COVID-19 pandemic: Resilience matters. Arch Gerontol Geriatr 2020;89:104124.
14. Voysey LR, El Sahly HM, Essink B, et al. Efficacy and safety of the mRNA-1273 SARS-CoV-2 vaccine. N Engl J Med 2021;384(5):403–16.
15. Voysey M, Clemens SAC, Madhi SA, et al. Safety and efficacy of the ChAdOx1 nCoV-19 vaccine (AZD1222) against SARS-CoV-2: an interim analysis of four randomised controlled trials in Brazil, South Africa, and the UK. Lancet 2021; 397(10269):99–111.

16. Farge G, de Wazières B, Raude J, et al. The health professional's view on the inclusion of age in the recommendations for pneumococcal vaccination: results of a cross-sectional survey in France. Geriatrics (Basel) 2021;7(1):4.
17. Wu Q, Dudley MZ, Chen X, et al. Evaluation of the safety profile of COVID-19 vaccines: a rapid review. BMC Med 2021;19(1):173.
18. Osterholm MT, Kelley NS, Sommer A, et al. Efficacy and effectiveness of influenza vaccines: a systematic review and meta-analysis. Lancet Infect Dis 2012;12(1): 36–44.
19. Ciabattini A, Nardini C, Santoro F, et al. Vaccination in the elderly: the challenge of immune changes with aging. Semin Immunol 2018;40:83–94.
20. Iuliano AD, Roguski KM, Chang HH, et al. Estimates of global seasonal influenza-associated respiratory mortality: a modelling study. Lancet 2018;391(10127): 1285–300.
21. Andrew MK, Bowles SK, Pawelec G, et al. Influenza vaccination in older adults: recent innovations and practical applications. Drugs Aging 2019;36(1):29–37.
22. Cunningham AL, McIntyre P, Subbarao K, et al. Vaccines for older adults. BMJ 2021;372:n188. Published 2021 Feb 22.
23. Rondy M, El Omeiri N, Thompson MG, et al. Effectiveness of influenza vaccines in preventing severe influenza illness among adults: a systematic review and meta-analysis of test-negative design case-control studies. J Infect 2017;75(5):381–94.
24. Nichols MK, Andrew MK, Hatchette TF, et al. Influenza vaccine effectiveness to prevent influenza-related hospitalizations and serious outcomes in Canadian adults over the 2011/12 through 2013/14 influenza seasons: a pooled analysis from the Canadian Immunization Research Network (CIRN) serious outcomes surveillance (SOS Network). Vaccine 2018;36(16):2166–75.
25. Lewnard JA, Cobey S. Immune history and influenza vaccine effectiveness. Vaccines (Basel) 2018;6(2):28. Published 2018 May 21.
26. Lee JKH, Lam GKL, Shin T, et al. Efficacy and effectiveness of high-dose influenza vaccine in older adults by circulating strain and antigenic match: an updated systematic review and meta-analysis. Vaccine 2021;39(Suppl 1):A24–35.
27. Oxman MN, Levin MJ, Johnson GR, et al. A vaccine to prevent herpes zoster and postherpetic neuralgia in older adults. N Engl J Med 2005;352(22):2271–84.
28. Oxman MN, Harbecke R, Koelle DM. Clinical usage of the adjuvanted herpes zoster subunit vaccine (HZ/su): Revaccination of recipients of live attenuated zoster vaccine and coadministration with a seasonal influenza vaccine. J Infect Dis 2017;216(11):1329–33.
29. Arvin AM. Humoral and cellular immunity to varicella-zoster virus: an overview. J Infect Dis 2008;197(Suppl 2):S58–60.
30. Dendouga N, Fochesato M, Lockman L, et al. Cell-mediated immune responses to a varicella-zoster virus glycoprotein E vaccine using both a TLR agonist and QS21 in mice. Vaccine 2012;30(20):3126–35.
31. Lal H, Cunningham AL, Godeaux O, et al. Efficacy of an adjuvanted herpes zoster subunit vaccine in older adults. N Engl J Med 2015;372(22):2087–96.
32. Cunningham AL, Lal H, Kovac M, et al. Efficacy of the herpes zoster subunit vaccine in adults 70 years of age or older. N Engl J Med 2016;375(11):1019–32.
33. Juergens C, de Villiers PJ, Moodley K, et al. Safety and immunogenicity of 13-valent pneumococcal conjugate vaccine formulations with and without aluminum phosphate and comparison of the formulation of choice with 23-valent pneumococcal polysaccharide vaccine in elderly adults: a randomized open-label trial. Hum Vaccin Immuno Ther 2014;10(5):1343–53.

34. Wagner A, Weinberger B. Vaccines to prevent infectious diseases in the older population: immunological challenges and future perspectives. Front Immunol 2020;11:717. Published 2020 Apr 23.

35. Matanock A, Lee G, Gierke R, et al. Use of 13-valent pneumococcal conjugate vaccine and 23-valent pneumococcal polysaccharide vaccine among adults aged ≥65 Years: updated recommendations of the advisory committee on immunization practices. MMWR Morb Mortal Wkly Rep 2019;68(46):1069–75.

36. Sharma O, Sultan AA, Ding H, et al. A review of the progress and challenges of developing a vaccine for COVID-19. Front Immunol 2020;11:585354.

37. Awadasseid A, Wu Y, Tanaka Y, et al. Current advances in the development of SARS-CoV-2 vaccines. Int J Biol Sci 2021;17(1):8–19.

38. Mathew S, Faheem M, Hassain NA, et al. Platforms exploited for SARS-CoV-2 vaccine development. Vaccines (Basel) 2020;9(1):11.

39. Funk CD, Laferrière C, Ardakani A. A snapshot of the global race for vaccines targeting SARS-CoV-2 and the COVID-19 pandemic. Front Pharmacol 2020;11:937.

40. Li Y, Tenchov R, Smoot J, et al. A comprehensive review of the global efforts on COVID-19 vaccine development. ACS Cent Sci 2021;7(4):512–33.

41. Rawat K, Kumari P, Saha L. COVID-19 vaccine: a recent update in pipeline vaccines, their design and development strategies. Eur J Pharmacol 2021;892:173751.

42. WHO—COVID19 vaccine tracker. Available at. https://covid19.trackvaccines.org/agency/who/. Accessed January 28, 2022.

43. Jackson LA, Anderson EJ, Rouphael NG, et al. An mRNA vaccine against SARS-CoV-2 - preliminary report. N Engl J Med 2020;383(20):1920–31.

44. Umakanthan S, Chattu VK, Ranade AV, et al. A rapid review of recent advances in diagnosis, treatment and vaccination for COVID-19. AIMS Public Health 2021;8(1):137–53.

45. Lazarus JV, Ratzan SC, Palayew A, et al. A global survey of potential acceptance of a COVID-19 vaccine. Nat Med 2021;27(2):225–8.

46. Sallam M. COVID-19 vaccine hesitancy worldwide: a concise systematic review of vaccine acceptance rates. Vaccines (Basel) 2021;9(2):160.

47. Billah MA, Miah MM, Khan MN. Reproductive number of coronavirus: a systematic review and meta-analysis based on global level evidence. PLoS One 2020;15(11):e0242128.

48. Anderson RM, Vegvari C, Truscott J, et al. Challenges in creating herd immunity to SARS-CoV-2 infection by mass vaccination. Lancet 2020;396(10263):1614–6.

49. Britton T, Ball F, Trapman P. A mathematical model reveals the influence of population heterogeneity on herd immunity to SARS-CoV-2. Science 2020;369(6505):846–9.

50. Clinic Mayo. US COVID-19 vaccine tracker: see your state's progress. Available at: https://www.mayoclinic.org/coronavirus-covid-19/vaccine-tracker. Accessed January 28, 2022.

51. National flu and COVID-19 surveillance reports: 2021 to 2022 season: 16 December 2021 (week 50). Available at: https://www.gov.uk/government/statistics/national-flu-and-covid-19-surveillance-reports-2021-to-2022-season. Accessed January 28, 2022.

52. Troiano G, Nardi A. Vaccine hesitancy in the era of COVID-19. Public Health 2021;194:245–51.

53. Aw J, Seng JJB, Seah SSY, et al. COVID-19 vaccine hesitancy-a scoping review of literature in high-income countries. Vaccines (Basel). 2021;9(8):900.

54. Biswas MR, Alzubaidi MS, Shah U, et al. A scoping review to find out worldwide COVID-19 vaccine hesitancy and its underlying determinants. Vaccines (Basel) 2021;9(11):1243.
55. Cesari M, Vellas B. Older persons "Lost" to the COVID-19 vaccination: where are they? J Frailty Aging 2021;10(4):308–9.
56. Gallè F, Sabella EA, Roma P, et al. Acceptance of COVID-19 vaccination in the elderly: a cross-sectional study in southern Italy. Vaccines (Basel) 2021;9(11): 1222.
57. Strategy to achieve global Covid-19 vaccination by mid-20222021. World Health Organization. Available at: https://www.who.int/publications/m/item/strategy-to-achieve-global-covid-19-vaccination-by-mid-2022. Accessed December 25 2021.
58. Chakraborty C, Sharma AR, Bhattacharya M, et al. All nations must prioritize the COVID-19 vaccination program for elderly adults urgently. Aging Dis 2021;12(3): 688–90.
59. Framework for decision-making: implementation of mass vaccination campaigns in the context of COVID-19: interim guidance. World Health Organization. Available at: https://apps.who.int/iris/handle/10665/332159. Accessed May 22 2021.
60. Overview of the implementation of COVID-19 vaccination strategies and deployment plans in the EU/EEa. European centre for disease prevention and control at: https://www.ecdc.europa.eu/en/publications-data/overview-implementation-covid-19-vaccination-strategies-and-deployment-plans. Accessed January 31, 2022.
61. Hasan T, Beardsley J, Marais BJ, et al. The implementation of mass-vaccination against SARS-CoV-2: a systematic review of existing strategies and guidelines. Vaccines (Basel) 2021;9(4):326.
62. Chakraborty C, Sharma AR, Bhattacharya M, et al. COVID-19 vaccines and vaccination program for aging adults. Eur Rev Med Pharmacol Sci 2021; 25(21):6719–30.
63. Privor-Dumm LA, Poland GA, Barratt J, et al. A global agenda for older adult immunization in the COVID-19 era: a roadmap for action. Vaccine 2021;39(37): 5240–50.
64. Soiza RL, Scicluna C, Thomson EC. Efficacy and safety of COVID-19 vaccines in older people. Age Ageing 2021;50(2):279–83.
65. Prendki V, Tau N, Avni T, et al. A systematic review assessing the underrepresentation of elderly adults in COVID-19 trials. BMC Geriatr 2020;20(1): 538. Published 2020 Dec 20.
66. Antonelli Incalzi R, Trevisan C, Del Signore S, et al. Are vaccines against COVID-19 tailored to the most vulnerable people? Vaccine 2021;39(17):2325–7.
67. Wang X. Safety and efficacy of the BNT162b2 mRNA Covid-19 vaccine. N Engl J Med 2021;384(16):1577–8.
68. Hewitt J, Carter B, Vilches-Moraga A, et al. The effect of frailty on survival in patients with COVID-19 (COPE): a multicentre, European, observational cohort study. Lancet Public Health 2020;5(8):e444–51.
69. Tut G, Lancaster T, Krutikov M, et al. Profile of humoral and cellular immune responses to single doses of BNT162b2 or ChAdOx1 nCoV-19 vaccines in residents and staff within residential care homes (VIVALDI): an observational study. Lancet Healthy Longev 2021;2(9):e544–53.
70. Wyller TB, Kittang BR, Ranhoff AH, et al. Nursing home deaths after COVID-19 vaccination. Dødsfall i sykehjem etter covid-19-vaksine. Tidsskr Nor Laegeforen 2021;141.

71. Harrison J, Berry S, Mor V, et al. Somebody like Me": understanding COVID-19 vaccine hesitancy among staff in skilled nursing facilities. J Am Med Dir Assoc 2021;22(6):1133–7.

72. Salmerón Ríos S, Mas Romero M, Cortés Zamora EB, et al. Immunogenicity of the BNT162b2 vaccine in frail or disabled nursing home residents: COVID-A study. J Am Geriatr Soc 2021;69(6):1441–7.

73. Shrotri M, Krutikov M, Palmer T, et al. Vaccine effectiveness of the first dose of ChAdOx1 nCoV-19 and BNT162b2 against SARS-CoV-2 infection in residents of long-term care facilities in England (VIVALDI): a prospective cohort study. Lancet Infect Dis 2021;21(11):1529–38.

74. Kahn R, Holmdahl I, Reddy S, et al. Mathematical modeling to inform vaccination strategies and testing approaches for COVID-19 in nursing homes. Clin Infect Dis 2021;74(4):597-603. ciab517.

75. Domi M, Leitson M, Gifford D, et al. The BNT162b2 vaccine is associated with lower new COVID-19 cases in nursing home residents and staff. J Am Geriatr Soc 2021;69(8):2079–89.

76. Teran RA, Walblay KA, Shane EL, et al. Postvaccination SARS-CoV-2 infections among skilled nursing facility residents and staff members - Chicago, Illinois, December. Am J Transpl 2021;21(6):2290–7.

77. Palermo S. Covid-19 pandemic: maximizing future vaccination treatments considering aging and frailty. Front Med (Lausanne) 2020;7:558835.

78. Feikin D, Higdon MM, Abu-Raddad LJ, et al. Duration of effectiveness of vaccines against SARS-CoV-2 infection and COVID-19 disease: results of a systematic review and meta-regression. Lancet 2022;399(10328):924-944 (Pre-print).

79. WHO SAGE Roadmap for prioritizing uses of COVID-19 vaccines. World Health Organization. Available at: https://www.who.int/publications/i/item/who-sage-roadmap-for-prioritizing-uses-of-covid-19-vaccines. Accessed January 21, 2022.

80. Atmar RL, Lyke KE, Deming ME, et al. Homologous and heterologous Covid-19 booster vaccinations. N Engl J Med 2022;386:1046-1057.

81. Sablerolles RSG, Rietdijk WJR, Goorhuis A, et al. Immunogenicity and reactogenicity of vaccine boosters after Ad26.COV2.S priming. N Engl J Med 2022; 386(10):951-963.

82. Costa Clemens SA, Weckx L, Clemens R, et al. Heterologous versus homologous COVID-19 booster vaccination in previous recipients of two doses of CoronaVac COVID-19 vaccine in Brazil (RHH-001): a phase 4, non-inferiority, single blind, randomised study. Lancet 2022;S0140-6736(22):00094–100.

83. Arbel R, Hammerman A, Sergienko R, et al. BNT162b2 vaccine booster and mortality due to Covid-19. N Engl J Med 2021;385(26):2413–20.

84. Bar-On YM, Goldberg Y, Mandel M, et al. Protection against Covid-19 by BNT162b2 booster across age groups. N Engl J Med 2021;385(26):2421–30.

85. CDC COVID-19 Vaccine Booster Shots. Center for disease control and prevention. Available at: https://www.cdc.gov/coronavirus/2019-ncov/vaccines/booster-shot.html. Accessed January 21, 2022.

86. Shakespeare T, Ndagire F, Seketi QE. Triple jeopardy: disabled people and the COVID-19 pandemic. Lancet 2021;397(10282):1331–3.

87. Andrew MK, Schmader KE, Rockwood K, et al. Considering frailty in SARS-CoV-2 vaccine development: how geriatricians can assist. Clin Interv Aging 2021;16: 731–8.

88. Andrew MK, McElhaney JE. Age and frailty in COVID-19 vaccine development. Lancet 2021;396(10267):1942–4.

Moving?

Make sure your subscription moves with you!

To notify us of your new address, find your **Clinics Account Number** (located on your mailing label above your name), and contact customer service at:

Email: journalscustomerservice-usa@elsevier.com

800-654-2452 (subscribers in the U.S. & Canada)
314-447-8871 (subscribers outside of the U.S. & Canada)

Fax number: 314-447-8029

Elsevier Health Sciences Division
Subscription Customer Service
3251 Riverport Lane
Maryland Heights, MO 63043

*To ensure uninterrupted delivery of your subscription, please notify us at least 4 weeks in advance of move.

Printed and bound by CPI Group (UK) Ltd, Croydon, CR0 4YY

03/10/2024

01040470-0017